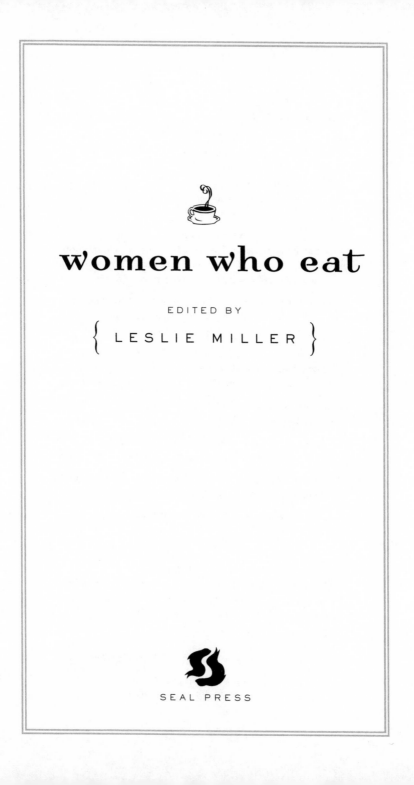

women who eat

EDITED BY

{ LESLIE MILLER }

SEAL PRESS

Women Who Eat: A NEW GENERATION ON THE GLORY OF FOOD
© 2003 by Leslie Miller

Published by
Seal Press
An Imprint of Avalon Publishing Group Incorporated
245 West 17th Street, 11th Floor
New York, NY 10011

Library of Congress Cataloging-in-Publication Data

Women who eat
p. cm.
ISBN 1-58005-092-1 (pbk.)
1. Food writing. 2. Women Food writers—United States. 3. Cookery.
TX643.W65 2003
641.5'082—dc22   2003057339

9   8   7   6   5   4   3   2   1

Designed by Pauline Neuwirth, Neuwirth & Associates, Inc.

Printed in the United States of America
Distributed by Publishers Group West

contents

 indicates essays that contain recipes.

contents

contents

contents

for Atticus

acknowledgments

F IRST OF ALL, thanks to all of the inspiring women—living and no—throughout literary culinary history who helped shape the gastronomical me, as it were. You are intrepid role models each of you—joyful, sybaritic, and wise.

Thanks to my officemates and officemates in absentia who believed in this project—Ingrid, Tina, Will, and Nate—and who suffered through my (I thought) stifled bouts of authorial mania. Thank you to my patient, brilliant editor, Christina, for helpful manuscript guidance and for those decadent long talks about meals and restaurants conducted in lieu of actual editorial work. Thank you to Jessica for crossing my t's and dotting my i's. Thanks to Troy for teaching me how to clean squid, among other gifts. And thanks of course to the splendid women whose work fills these pages—each of you made this project a success and a joy.

acknowledgments

Thanks to my family: my mother, who imparted a love of all things grown by one's own hand: peanuts and bronze fennel, warty cucumbers and strawberries; my father, a devoted enophile who first taught me as a young girl how to open Champagne (and pour it correctly), and also taught me that life is too short to drink bad wine; and my brothers—a carnivorous, loquacious bunch of hunters, good eaters, and exacting cooks who make every Thanksgiving a three-fold reenactment of Jacques and Julia in the kitchen. Thanks to Grams, who among other things first taught me to drive, bake, and make watermelon pickles. Thanks to my aunts for frying and powdering *fattigmann* with me, and for showing me that the rough handling of bread dough is indeed therapeutic.

And for my beloved Matt Hendel, and charming young son Atticus, who, by the age of one, has eaten, among other foods, beef Wellington, *doro wat,* and as many spring rolls as he has ever been given—a million thanks for supporting and enduring my many hours holed up in my office, for the baths given alone and bedtime stories missed. I promise you years of good meals in exchange.

introduction

"**Y**OU MUST TELL me all your favorite books, then! What was the last novel you read?"

My son had an appointment with the pediatrician, and he, the pediatrician, had discovered I edit books for a living. His was the first question that usually comes up when I discuss my job with folks not in the business (in Seattle the publishing industry still seems somewhat glamorous to most). Having been ordained an "expert," they are sure I can point them to either some obscure literary classic or the new Tolstoy, an undiscovered gem—like one of Calvin Trillin's found food carts under a New York City overpass or an honest, cheap mechanic. I struggled to remember the most recent novel I'd read and liked, and while we debated the dubious merits of *The Corrections* over a naked, writhing child, I mused on what my honest answer would have been.

My favorite books? There is the self-published Ethiopian cookbook with the photo of the proud matriarch and a recipe for *berbere* that begins, "Take ten pounds of bird's eye chilies, wash them, then let them dry in the sun for two days . . ." Or Elizabeth David on the merits of fresh nutmeg, a kernel of which she kept in her purse. There is *Kimchi: A Korean Health Food,* written by two Korean-American home economists, replete with color photographs and recipes for "soothingly tasty" radish or "refreshingly tangy" oyster *kimchi.* A 1926 tome on composed hotel salads that conjures visions of lunches with the Fitzgeralds, and the *Paul Prudhomme Family Cookbook* within whose pages a sprawling, food-loving, sharecropping family comes to life and the recipe for the enigmatic "Turducken"—a chicken stuffed inside a duck stuffed inside a turkey—waits patiently for the day when my boning skills are honed and I've two days to spare and fifteen people to feed.

As the mother of a small boy my reading time is scant, and usually absorbed by the manuscripts heaped at my bedside; but my nightstand is also always littered with food magazines, food memoirs, and cookbooks that I shuffle from bedroom to kitchen to bedroom again. I've read more than a few novels over the last two decades of course, but the novels I remember most vividly still are children's books by authors like Roald Dahl and Wilson Rawls or Laura Ingalls Wilder—glorious stuff that enthralled me in grade school and continues to linger mostly because of the honest, painstaking descriptions of food: enormous ripe peaches and Toad in the Hole, cold cornbread and a first strawberry soda, salt pork and taffy made with store-bought sugar that refuses to stiffen in the hot afternoon air. Much like Harriet the Spy with her tomato sandwiches, as a young girl I holed up with these books beneath sycamore canopies and under beds, picking my way through sci-fi and mystery, adventure and history, by following a trail of literary breadcrumbs; a well-described meal connoted far more to me than any other expositor, taking me into New

York apartments and unsettled midwestern plains, the rough hills of the Ozark Mountains. And then, around the magical age of twelve, I discovered cookbooks.

As a young girl in a small town in the "other" Washington, *The Silver Palate* read like a thriller. Its East coast pretentiousness, its delicious fussiness—the breezy cataloguing of kosher foods and the best *cornichon,* goat cheeses rolled in ash and light yet elaborate meals for after the theater—who were these strange and wonderful people? And what of these strange and wonderful foods? It was then I began to make the connection between the magic of the kitchen and descriptions of food—I pored over my grandmother's spidery script on stained index cards detailing preparations for Parker House rolls and watermelon pickles, marveled at the then utterly tony and unfathomable *Gourmet* magazine and the elaborate French meals eaten by the glitterati in New York, and began to experiment my way through my mother's cookbooks—both *Silver Palate* volumes, Julia Child, and an illustrated book of Chinese cooking. That Easter I unearthed a photograph in a women's magazine of a stunning centerpiece—a ham *en croûte,* coated with duxelles and wrapped in layers of phyllo. As it was set upon the table and all set to tittering over the crispy, golden hunk of mushroom-scented pork, I absorbed the adulation like sustenance. I was hooked.

Yet as I entered adolescence and then early adulthood, while I continued to perfect my challah and experimented with *ma pao tofu* and chicken Kiev, I watched my food obsession fall out of favor. Teen girls these days are coached in ways of lip gloss, not in the joys of conquering an emulsion sauce. The message to me was clear: Young women did not debate the merits of whipped egg whites in their waffle batters or put "new KitchenAid" on their Christmas lists. Women didn't cook as much as they prepared meals, grudgingly, and once they were married, for families not for fun. Women didn't eat, they dieted, and talked rapaciously about everything they weren't eating. Women didn't read cookbooks, they read fashion magazines, or Marxist theory, but you were in one camp or the other, and neither gave so much as a nod to the kitchen. How boring. I wagered even Marxists eat, and cook, collectively perhaps, but even so. As I baked my way through college and celebrity-chef culture exploded around me, I tired even more of the pop-culture cult of women and their bodies, of women and their diets, of the polar extremes of *Mademoiselle* or Marx.

After a while, I'd had enough. If conventional wisdom dictated that women—not kitchen-captive Betty Crockers but freewheeling, careered, post–Mary Tyler Moores—did not care about food aside from cutting coupons for Wednesday night's roast and translating Weight Watchers points, then disproving this notion would require some unconventional thinking. To be sure, the last decade or so has seen the publication of volumes of women's memoirs—brilliant accounts of love affairs with food by gourmet goddesses from Ruth Reichl to Madeleine Kamman. I devoured them one by one and each proved a temporary tonic for my fever—but I wanted more.

I wanted to read too about women like me—women obsessed and in love with all things gastronomical, who hadn't necessarily translated that passion into a livelihood. I wanted to eavesdrop on a conversation—a conversation between women, not about low carb but about last night's buttered noodles, or the first favas in spring, or mutti's meatballs, or the long simmered greens of their childhood—but I was completely unprepared for how many other women wanted to join in. In preparing this collection, women from every corner of North America, some who cooked and some who couldn't boil water, professional chefs and lawyers and stay-at-home moms, women as young as twenty and well into their seventies sent in their stories. And every woman who wrote in said thank you, thank you for "allowing" me to write about food! I began to suspect that if women were allowed to concentrate on food as much as they wished, nothing else would get done. No laundry, no defending clients, no writing or running the world. Just women sautéing and steaming, fingering voluptuous produce and boning out chickens, and, more importantly, eating.

I am a devoted aficionada of the contemporary culinary scene, don't get me wrong, but so much of popular food culture is about glamour—postmodern restaurant trends, "foreign" culinary exotica from far-off lands, or popular mad food scientists sacrificing dozens of roosters in the name of the perfect cassoulet. What's often left out of the popular food-writing canon forms the most intimate side of our eating habits—our cravings, what we eat straight from the pot, the dishes that transport us back to different places or times, or truly signify home. Above all, *Women Who Eat* isn't a glamorous collection of food writing but an honest, earthy, meaty one, replete with dirty dishes and sex and fat and shortcuts, farmers' markets and dinner parties and even our favorite restaurants, those that comfort us rather than dazzle us with presentation or a secret phone line for reservations.

More than a few of these essays feature our mothers or grandmothers (and a father or two)—who taught us how to cook and eat simply by allowing us into the kitchen, who first juggled families and careers and cooking, and, despite the cream-of-mushroom-soup years, managed to create daughters in love with food or cooking or both. These essays also feature children—some of them the authors themselves who once upon a time swapped paper lunch bags of homemade *aloo gobi* for the American anonymity of canned corn and fishsticks, or learned by osmosis the art of entertaining, or were raised on food pulled up from the sea or grown in backyard gardens and put up in sparkling Mason jars or earthenware crocks. Without being trendy, these writers discover for themselves the benefits and joys of knowing where their food comes from and engaging in the delicious relationships that can form between those who grow our vegetables or make our cheese or raise our beef and those who prepare and consume it with a newfound reverence. Some reject the rigidity and formality of haute cuisine in favor of cleaner, brighter flavors or the comfort and warmth of frugal, dowdy foods like humble sauerkraut. Other women discover what it is to literally become food—to nurture a child growing within or create milk to sustain a newborn. One writer even challenges the very notion of autocannibalism with a need born of a postpartum body.

These women discover the range of cultures in America, and relate lessons learned by different peoples: the proper way to fry an egg—the *Thai* way—or the African lesson that food, in and of itself, is a gift. They understand food as a conduit of heritage and tradition embodied in Jewish mandelbrot, or midwestern casseroles, or a fifteen-course Sicilian feast, and dismiss those who assume that women today fear rather than revere food, "heat" instead of cook, that the intricate lessons of the kitchens from generations of women before were destroyed by microwaves and takeout. Some are still learning—some can't make rice or are stymied by the simplest of recipes—but still they continue to cook. In my world, ultimately even the novices will prevail, and those who can't cook will still enjoy the fruits of the labor of others and join the legion of women, the majority of women, the women who eat.

LESLIE MILLER
SEATTLE, 2003

big night, *or* wound a sicilian, pay through the mouth

{ CAMILLE CUSUMANO }

MY SISTER GRACE—who is my junior by a year and four days—and I were once each other's shadow. We answered to each other's name, covered for each other's "crimes," and generally practiced *omertà*—before we could even pronounce this Sicilian word for the code of silence. Then things changed. Grace took a husband, a big house, and had kids. I took to the road in search of myself.

A few years ago, my sister, who never shared my desperate need to escape New Jersey, expressed interest in accompanying me on my world travels. I suggested she join me on a trip to Sicily, home to our forebears, during which I planned to lodge in hermitages open to lay travelers. She jumped at the chance.

By the time we reached Catania, the province dominated by the active volcano, Mt. Etna, it was apparent how set we were in our different ways. Grace enjoyed sleeping late, while I was up early. She liked lots of cappuccino stops, I liked to keep moving. She wanted shopping and beach sitting, but I insisted on the pursuit of monastic settings.

The one exception to our contrasting time management was food. We were bred into the soulful necessity of the well-composed feast. Our Sicilian grandparents put forth even the humblest meal— crusty bread, sweet butter, and wine, say—with the same reverence a priest bestows upon Holy Communion. Food wasn't just sacred. It was *good*. We were fed greens like chard, broccoli rabe, dandelions, and cardoons, cooked fresh from our grandparents' gardens. We ate mounds of hand-rolled pasta, prepared in a variety of luscious ways, long before it was fashionable in America.

With hunger pangs uniting us one evening, we arrived at Acireale, a baroque town that sits on a sloping haunch of the moody firepit, Etna, over the Ionian Sea. We would spend the night in the eighteenth-century Franciscan monastery, San Biagio, amid cloisters, frescoes, lush gardens, statuary, and three ostriches.

On our way out for dinner, we passed a coarse-robed friar strolling the long halls. He jangled his ring of skeleton keys, reminding us that our lodging had a curfew. Yet we still had plenty of time to savor a long, slow dinner, Sicilian style. We ambled down the narrow back streets to the main thoroughfare, Via Vittorio Emanuele II, scrutinizing each and every restaurant. We were looking for signs—unpretentious lighting, paper tablecloths, men wearing bibs to guard against red splashes, dented metal pots on a hot stove, a plump grandmotherly type chanting a few bars of the melodious dialect, *Ven aca, sedi, mangia!* (Come here, sit, eat!)

With its cuisine (like its liturgy) founded on three farm products— wheat, olives, and grapes—Sicily doesn't lack for tempting menus. But we had been disappointed by a mediocre made-for-tourists meal the night before in Cefalù. I had ordered, assiduously in

Italian, the *polpo* (octopus), remembering my grandmother's delicious version stuffed with bread crumbs, cheese, and herbs, and steeped in tomato broth. Sadly, the vulcanized fiber laid before us was better suited for soling a shoe. We were determined not to repeat the experience.

We finally settled on Oste Scuro at Piazza Lionardo Vigo. It was not quite the snapshot of our grandparents' kitchens, but its alfresco terrace across from a floodlit cathedral was warm and inviting. We watched two handsome, well-heeled couples step from a shiny black limousine and vanish laughing into the shadowy interior of the restaurant. They exuded a certain glamour mixed with an easy sensuality.

As our eyes followed them, I asked Grace, "What do you think?"

"Let's give it a try," she said. I agreed, noticing that most patrons seemed to be Italian, not the Anglo tourists notorious for their lack of discriminating taste. I told the maitre d' in my best Italian—cobbled together from college courses and remembrance of words passed between Mom and Dad—that we wanted only to eat well, not like tourists as we had in Cefalù.

I began to expound on the previous night's rubbery octopus, but trailed off as I saw his face flush deeply, his eyes dart in the sign of the cross, his nostrils flare. What had I said?

I was raised in an expressive culture. My own mercurial father could display passion, anger, disappointment, and tenderness with a mere glance, and my sister and I translated his meaning the way a blind person reads Braille, or a fisherman reads the sea.

My complaining had vexed the man, stirring up animosity for us implacable tourists. *Perhaps we should leave,* I thought. But he took a deep breath, and with a dignified and ceremonial flourish ushered us to a table. "Sit," he ordered tersely. We obeyed like the dutiful girls we had once been in our traditional Sicilian family.

"What did you say?" whispered Grace, who had not missed the surfeit of climate changes in his face.

{3}

"I know what I said," I told her, still wondering if we should just bolt, "I'm not sure what he *heard*."

Presently, the maitre d' returned with two other men, one waiter and one dressed smartly in a suit. They had obviously been clued in that we were complainers. Our longed-for repast would be foiled again.

A carafe of red wine was set before us. After allowing us to briefly study the extensive menu, the three concluded that we should let them feed us. Their imperious tone told us not to object. A side serving table was set up next to ours. This lovely weekend evening had brought many diners to the popular Oste Scuro. Yet none seemed to be getting the attention we were receiving.

Oste Scuro's menu featured at least twenty different *antipasti,* representing every flavor of Sicily that has seduced discriminating palates since Archestrato di Gela wrote the first cookbook, *The Sweet Taste,* 400 years before Christ. Grace and I were served in slow procession tangy-sweet caponata, platters of fried eggplant, fresh creamy ricotta, buffalo-milk mozzarella, prosciutto, citrus and onion salad, broccoli rabe and wild fennel redolent of garlic and olive oil, conch tender as a first kiss, fire-roasted peppers. We took a few breaths and forked onto our plates *fritto misto* of artichokes and squid, frittata larded with pancetta, fresh fava beans and peas, and roasted potatoes with caramelized garlic toes.

Every taste sensation between earth and sun, from the pungent to the sweet to the sour, was laid upon our tongues. Generosity is nourishment in and of itself, and we would have felt sated, even if these dishes had been less phenomenal. To our astonished delight, more *antipasti* were set before us—marinated porcini, fresh sardines, mussels, shrimp, and sautéed calamari. We worked the goodness from each morsel like bees sucking nectar from flowers.

As the parade of dishes crowded the serving table near us I learned that the smartly dressed man regaling us was none other

than Oste Scuro owner Carmelo Muscolino, who has run the establishment for more than thirty years. The pride Muscolino takes in
his country's cooking was evidenced in these local ingredients, from
the fruits of sea and earth to the piquant kiss of garlic, fragrant
embrace of olive oil, and tingle of lemon.

"Don't look now," I said to Grace, "but one of the guys waiting on us is *il padrone* himself, master of the house."

"I'll kiss his ring," said Grace, smacking her lips, "his food is
fabulous."

"I'm afraid he'll kill the cook," I said, "if I tell him it's anything but."

Catania's specialties include the aromatic pasta Norma, a riga-
toni with tomatoes, fried eggplant, basil, and the sharp *ricotta salata*;
pasta cc'a mudica, made with toasted bread crumbs, olive oil, and
anchovies; *pasta cc'u trunzu*, with specially cultivated cabbage; and
pasta cc'u niuru, mantled in a dark, sweet mix of squid ink and tomatoes. We were served Oste Scuro's versions of each one, plentiful
enough to feed six people. Grace and I looked at each other. We
understood that to stop eating was tantamount to trampling the flag.

But with each delightful swallow, my eyes bulged. My waistline felt no more distinct than the middle of a bell pepper. The
taste of the food and the sheer abundance transported me back to
my childhood when not one of our parents' ten children dared leave
the table before cleaning his or her plate.

"Take small portions and eat very slowly," I advised Grace.

"Easy for you to say," she said, noticing that I would offer to
serve her first, filling her plate with more food than I then took.
I pushed the thought of the bill away. It loomed like an unreal
denouement in a Fellini film.

I began to understand how my cavalier criticism had desecrated
these Sicilians' cherished patrimony. They were ashamed of their
compatriot who had fed us so poorly that I had felt compelled to

broadcast it. The abundance and diversity of food served us—with nary a hint of fawning—was an implicit gag order. We accepted the "penance" for my blasphemy.

The four *paste* were delicious, perfectly *al dente* and balanced in the pairing of chewy and tender textures and the mixtures of flavors—sweet, salty, robust, mild, aromatic. Each attested that the true genius of Sicilian cooking is in the use of honest, fresh ingredients mingled in imaginative ways. I wanted to convey my innate understanding of this ancient alchemy to our waiter, but he was not interested in small talk. He nodded to the maitre d' who came by, smiled, and asked, "How is everything?"

"Extraordinary! Superb!" we assured him too eagerly.

"Bene," he said and told us to follow him. We stood, not without difficulty, and followed him inside the restaurant where we all leaned over a case of silver and iridescent fish on ice. He asked us to choose which we wanted, and when he saw the clouded look on our faces, pointed to a five-pound red snapper and asked, "Will this one do?"

"There's more?" asked Grace, panicky.

"Uhh . . . *sì* . . . of course . . ." I answered wistfully. I'd never been humbled by food in quite this way.

"How would you like it?" he asked.

"*To go*, tell him," said my sister who was on her first trip abroad. How to explain to her, whose mores have been steadfastly shaped in north Jersey, that she was no longer in Hoboken. I felt her eyes egging me to request that doggy bag.

"Grigliata?" he asked.

"Sì, sì," I mumbled. Grilled snapper it would be.

Back in our seats, I felt like a character in Jean Genet's theater of the absurd, uncertain of which side of the playwright's master-slave equation we represented. We sipped wine to revive our long-gone appetites for the fish course, and I refrained from telling Grace that *oste scuro* translates to "dark host." My thoughts grew even darker as I recalled that the thick menu included many types of *carne*, from rabbit and pork to veal scaloppini and famous Florentine Chianina beef, all of which I ordinarily love.

The snapper arrived. Discreetly, I loosened my belt two notches. Grace grabbed the serving utensils and served me the larger portion. "Hey, look!" I exclaimed. "Over there, that handsome man is staring at you!" I shoveled food from my plate back into hers as she turned. Of course, she didn't fall for that old gag, but the comic relief was welcome—even if it hurt to laugh. We were drunk, not on wine, but on food.

The snapper was meltingly sweet and moist, and we washed it down with more goblets of the rugged Catanese wine. Another platter arrived. It contained beautiful fresh fruit, including loquats, the sweet, white-fleshed Mediterranean fruit that would be criminal to pass up in Sicily. Just as I expelled the last of their mahogany pits, three different pastries appeared. I had always admired the Arabs' legacy to Sicily—an inventive finessing of almonds, pistachios, chocolate, sugar, eggs, and ricotta into an array of delectable *dolci*—until that moment. But we worked through the meal's crowning opulence like the actors with their death wish in *La Grande Bouffe*, even as the waiter posited a surreal trio of liqueurs—*limoncello*, *arancello*, and *cioccolato*—in front of us.

Tears filled our eyes and we pondered the existential question of whether we'd gone to heaven or hell. About the time the espresso arrived, we scared up the courage to ask our waiter to please bring a check—any check.

"*Ma, perché avete fretta?* (What's the hurry?)" he asked. You must try our gelato next. "*E fatto in casa.*"

"No, please! We love homemade gelato! Right, Grace?" I said, vaguely aware that my shrill tone belied my words. Grace wrung her hands. And then, in my desperation, I remembered some received wisdom, the one thing in Sicily that might trump their need to compensate their wounded pride—a woman's chaste reputation.

"*Signore,*" I begged, standing to block the way of our "dark host" to the kitchen that held our torture and delight. "We are lodging at San Biagio. They lock the doors at midnight. It's quarter to twelve—we must get back—or we'll have to sleep in the streets."

My plea magically triggered the evening's anti-climax. Our check arrived within minutes. It would be astronomical. We didn't care. Oh, we would pay anything for the pleasure of waddling away from that wonderful restaurant. But the full bill was only 158,000 lire, about $75 for two of us.

Ecstatic at the unexpectedly low total, I offered to treat Grace. It was a small price to pay for lessons learned on both our accounts. While I imparted a modicum of traveling etiquette to my younger sister (for instance, there is no Italian word for "doggy bag"), we both learned that one must also be prepared for the dark host. He could be lurking just behind the next *prezzo fisso* menu. Next time, my sister and I will remember what to do: *omertà.*

making tapioca

{ CHERYL STRAYED }

I DIDN'T COOK for men. I didn't cook. Especially for
men. But I loved him and he loved tapioca and making it became
my secret mission.

Tapioca pudding doesn't come easy. I'm not talking about imi-
tation stuff. I'm talking starting off with those hard pearls and your
job is to make them soft. Soft, but not too soft or the whole thing
will fall apart.

He held my hand as we walked the streets of Portland, Oregon.
We pointed out the houses we liked and spoke to the cats who watched
us from the porches. It was then that he told me about tapioca. He'd
had a grandmother from Sweden. Her name was Tekla and she didn't
speak English. What she did was have him sit in a chair in the kitchen
while she made him tapioca pudding. This was back when he was
six, seven, eight, in the years his parents were splitting up. She gave
him the whole bowl and encouraged him to eat it. And he did—the

whole thing. He ate and ate and she watched him eat and smiled when he made little sounds to himself, moans of pleasure.

I want to make you do that, I thought. Not from sex, but from something else. From me. From tapioca.

I didn't live with him yet. I lived with seven people I didn't know in a giant warehouse in the middle of which was a dark kitchen. None of the people were around when I was. But the mice were. They leapt from the shelves onto the counter or scuttled along the baseboards. This terrified me so I stood on a stool, squatting down over the stove to stir the tapioca.

A white bird flying away, he said. That's what I see when we finish making love. A white bird flying away.

I tasted the first batch. It occurred to me that I didn't know what I was getting into. I couldn't be exactly sure what tapioca pudding was supposed to taste like in the first place. I was not at that point a connoisseur of tapioca. There were lumps. Lumps with a hardness in the middle of them.

I tried again: the same thing.

I'm nobody's grandmother, I thought. The last thing I need to know is how to make a decent bowl of tapioca pudding. And who is he anyway?

I painted the walls of my section of the warehouse jet black. I read good books. I went to movies with him, museums; I roasted cloves of garlic and fresh red peppers and tossed them into angel hair pasta for dinner. I squeezed the fresh juice from grapefruits in the mornings after we'd finished making love.

Once he looked at me and made a circle in the air with his finger. What is that? I asked. It's how I am when I am with you, he said. It's what you are to me.

I tried again. This tapioca was clearly wrong—watery and bland, more a soup than a pudding. His birthday came and the tapioca

I had planned to surprise him with was fed to the dog who had stood by to beg for treats and chase the mice away.

Why make tapioca? I thought. There are plenty of other things in the world to eat. There are bananas and chocolate bars, sautéed wild mushrooms and baked potatoes, bagels and tomato soup. But then I thought of him leaning over the bowl and making that sound. That sound I elicited when I gave him an orgasm. That same sound, but not from sex. The sound of sex and also something else. I wanted to hear him do that. I wanted to be the one to make him.

I cooked another batch.

I stirred. I prayed.

I set the bowl on the table and watched it cool. It settled into a thick pale mass. It sparkled and congealed in the bowl. This was the tapioca I had been wanting all along. I covered the bowl with a plastic lid and wrapped the whole thing in purple tissue paper, tied a ribbon around it and drove to his house. It was afternoon, a cool day in April. I bent to set the bowl of tapioca on his doorstep. There was a heft to it, a weight like that of a body, a thing of one piece, the wings of a white bird flying away.

old-fashioned tapioca pudding

1 cup tapioca pearls

3 cups milk

3 cups heavy whipping cream

1 T. vanilla extract

1 cup sugar

4 egg yolks

4 egg whites

dash of salt

Cover the tapioca with water and soak at least four hours. Drain. Mix milk, cream, vanilla extract, and softened tapioca in a large pot. Cook over low heat, stirring every five minutes, until tapioca pearls are transparent, approximately one hour. Beat the egg yolks. Combine egg yolks, sugar, and salt, then add to the tapioca mixture slowly. Simmer, stirring constantly until the mixture is well combined and begins to thicken, five to ten minutes. Remove from heat. Beat the egg whites stiff and then fold them into the tapioca mixture. Pour into a bowl to cool. Chill in refrigerator before serving.

the way to a woman's heart

{ STEPHANIE SUSNJARA }

"I saw him even now going the way of all flesh, that is to say towards the kitchen."

—JOHN WEBSTER

𝓐 YOUNG WOMAN and a young man sit side by side on the edge of a rocky cliff. The sun has begun its descent, slipping behind distant mountain peaks, coloring the sky with ribbons of pink, purple, and gold. The woman cups the man's face in her hands, drawing him close. She takes her fingers and places something soft and creamy on his tongue. His eyes widen, but, before he can speak, the young woman presses her fingers against his lips.

"It's Montrachet—a goat cheese from France," she says.

The seduction continues. She feeds him baguette rounds topped with warm tarragon chicken salad, and strawberries dipped in chocolate. They wash it all down with a bottle of Gallo red table wine (although the woman considers herself a budding gourmet at twenty-one, she is still oblivious to fine vintages).

The sky is now dark and dusted with stars. Warmed by the food and wine, the two melt into each other's arms. The feasting has only just begun.

⁙

THE YOUNG MAN at that picnic eventually became my husband, and that is how I remember our first date. Between bites, I know we had intense, soul-baring conversation, but I can't remember a word of it. Instead, the seduction of taste buds—a wooing technique I inherited from my father—remains my most potent memory. Back then I fancied myself a food connoisseur, gently guiding this culinary virgin into a pleasure zone he had never even imagined.

Fifteen years later, it strokes my ego to remember the scene this way. Especially since my husband, Randy, has evolved into a passionate home chef who threatens to topple my long-held reign as the resident food goddess. Now he woos *me* by bathing jumbo shrimp in a honey-tangerine marinade, drizzling white truffle oil on mashed potatoes, and massaging ribeyes with cracked peppercorns, fresh rosemary, and garlic. On Friday nights, after we've put our three-year-old son to bed, Randy dims the lights, takes my hand, and leads me to the dining room. He disappears into the kitchen, leaving me at the table to relax and sip wine. Moments later he presents two plates. The other night it was roast duck in ginger sauce. Thin slices of the rich, juicy meat were fanned out around a perfect pyramid of jasmine-scented rice. A delicate mound of snow peas, glistening with sesame oil, provided a colorful balance. This artful presentation, known as "plating" in the restaurant biz, is a trick Randy picked up watching Food Network.

I'm still an avid cook, but I must admit, Randy has surpassed me when it comes to striving toward new culinary heights. I guess

I shouldn't complain about this role reversal. Until two generations ago, the men in my family never dreamed of donning aprons. Take my maternal grandfather Tony, a first-generation Sicilian-American doctor who ran a busy practice out of the first floor of the family brownstone in the Bushwick section of Brooklyn. He couldn't make toast and had no desire to try. The task of cooking was a domestic chore that belonged to my grandmother, a fact that became evident to me in my youth, on a hot afternoon in late July.

It was the summer of 1973. *American Graffiti* was playing at the box office and George Harrison was crooning "Give Me Love" on the radio. And like many Italian-American families, we never missed the ritual of Sunday dinner at my grandparents'. My grandfather, clad in plaid shorts and a white fishing hat, strolled into the dining room and took his place at the head of the table.

"Rose, get in here and sit down," he barked toward the kitchen.

My grandmother appeared in the doorway. She wiped her hands on a dishtowel. Her face was flushed with heat. Wisps of reddish brown hair had come unloose from her beehive hairdo. A floral-patterned sundress peeked out beneath her full-length apron. Her green eyes were fixed on my grandfather. "How's the sauce, Tony?"

Everyone turned toward my grandfather, who lifted a forkful of pasta. He paused a moment, savoring his power, before the fork disappeared inside his mouth.

"Too salty," he growled. My grandmother's smile was replaced with a look of defeat. She burst into tears, and ran into the kitchen.

The sauce didn't taste salty to me. It tasted perfect—thick and tomato-y, the best sauce in the world. Even at a young age, my grandmother's sauce filled me with pity for my non-Italian friends who thought spaghetti sauce came out of a jar.

Aunt Roseanne and my mother glared across the table at my grandfather. These sisters had grown weary of my grandfather's Old

World values and the oppression my grandmother put up with in her marriage. Across the country, women were bolting from the confines of the kitchen and entering the workforce. Aunt Roseanne worked full-time as an interior decorator. She wore strands of beads and platform shoes, strummed folk songs on the guitar, and dated guys with long hair. To my grandparents' dismay, she was thirty and *still* single. A suburban housewife, my mother wasn't quite as hip as Aunt Roseanne, but she didn't just tend the hearth, either. Mom spent countless hours fundraising for the local hospital and was working on her master's degree in volunteer management. Unlike her daughters, my grandmother never had the opportunity to pursue an identity beyond wife and mother.

"What?" my grandfather asked. He shrugged his shoulders and began attacking his plate. "Let's eat before this gets cold."

"You know, you're unbelievable," Aunt Roseanne said, slamming down her napkin. "Ma's been in there all day cooking for you."

My grandfather didn't even look up. Except for the clanking of silverware, we ate the remainder of the meal in silence.

My grandmother's tears startled me. By the age of nine I'd already spent many hours in her kitchen, elbows propped on her speckled linoleum table, watching as she stuffed spiky artichoke leaves with herbs and bread crumbs or rolled out fresh pizza dough. My grandmother made cooking seem effortless. She never relied on cookbooks. She always spoke with authority as she revealed her culinary secrets. "It's the Pecorino Romano," she'd say whenever I asked what gave her meatballs their savory flavor. She knew she was a great cook. I was shocked that my grandfather's little comment could bring her to tears, undermine the confidence I'd seen.

That Sunday afternoon in my grandparents' dining room, the politics of the home kitchen were revealed. For a woman of my grandmother's generation, cooking comprised a hefty portion of her marriage contract. She was simply expected to cook well. Every day of her married life, she was to have breakfast, lunch, and dinner on the table. My grandfather, who usually ate with his nose buried inside the newspaper, hurled complaints.

In my grandfather's eyes, cooking and serving food embodied the fundamental role of the housewife, and he wanted nothing to do with it. The only exception was barbecuing. Every Fourth of July he charred burgers, hot dogs, and long links of Italian sausage. My uncles and cousins would surround him in a football huddle, drinking beer and holding out slices of Italian bread for him to slap meat on. Outdoor cooking was the only acceptable form of home cooking for men of my grandfather's generation. Culinary icon James Beard helped fuel this macho American trend with the publication of *Cook It Outdoors* in 1941. All that fire and smoke made cooking a manly adventure, reminiscent of camping or combat.

I believe it was my grandfather's cold, unromantic attitude toward the home kitchen that attracted my mother to my father, a man who equated food with poetry. As a young man, Dad was a little ahead of his time when it came to taking his place in the kitchen.

·:·

MY PARENTS MET in 1959 while they were away at college on Philadelphia's Main Line. Dad was attending Villanova, a Catholic college for young men. A mile down the road, mom was cloistered with 500 other young girls at Rosemont College, another Catholic enclave. Early in their courtship, Dad invited my mother over for Sunday dinner. He lived with six other guys in a dilapidated row house on Lancaster Avenue, Villanova's main drag. Household responsibilities were divvied up, and my father volunteered to do all the cooking.

A first-generation American of Croatian and Czechoslovakian descent, Dad grew up in New York's Hell's Kitchen. He came from a long line of fabulous cooks—all women, of course. Nan Coric, his maternal grandmother from Bratislava, had fed him fork-tender pot roast, plump apple fritters, and the best fried chicken on earth. His Croatian Aunt Jenny made him smoked kielbasa with sauerkraut and homemade gnocchi—potato dumplings smothered in rich meat sauce. Dad loved to eat. He knew that if he wanted to continue eating well on his student budget, he'd have to cook himself.

Before he left for college, Dad began closely observing his female relatives in their kitchens. At school, he continued his culinary education, making trips to the library and used bookstores. He picked up volumes ranging from American housewife bibles *The Joy of Cooking* and *Betty Crocker's Picture Cook Book* to Brillat-Savarin's 1825 classic *The Physiology of Taste*, a book regarded as the first "food memoir," and *Larousse Gastronomique*, the vast encyclopedia of French and European cooking techniques, all of which he kept at his bedside and read late into the night. Every morning, while still lying in bed, Dad would stare up at the ceiling, smoking a cigarette and planning the evening menu, a habit he never lost.

When my mother arrived for that first dinner, she froze at the kitchen doorway. A mound of dirty bowls and utensils lay in the sink. Food was splattered on the counters, the walls, the ceiling. Tacked onto a kitchen cabinet was a note: Roaches Beware! My father's six-foot-three-inch frame was bent over the stove. His crewcut shone with sweat and a Lucky Strike with a long ash hung from his lips. Pots were going on all four burners. Dad was making gravy for a prime roast of beef, furiously stirring flour into a pan of meat drippings. Mom toyed with her pearl necklace until he looked up. The thick lenses of his black-rimmed glasses were fogged over with steam. "I hope you brought your appetite," he grinned, wiping his hands on the shirttails that hung out of his Bermuda shorts.

After they had drained the last glass of wine, my father took my mother's hand and led her to his bedroom. My mother expected to find his room plastered with posters of Marilyn Monroe, or Jane Russell. Instead, there was a large picture of a black-and-white collie hanging over his bed. He noticed her looking. "My dog Cindy," he said with pride. In the corner of the room, my mother noted large provolone cheeses, salamis, and prosciutto dangling from ceiling hooks. She breathed in their rich, smoky scent and was transported back to her Neapolitan grandmother's basement in Washington, D.C., where similar delicacies were stored along with bell jars of tomatoes, beans, eggplant, and vinegar peppers. What was this half-Croatian, half-Czechoslovakian guy doing with Italian goodies stashed in his room? Little did my mother realize that on the island of Olib off Croatia's Adriatic coast—where some of my father's ancestors originated—aged hams and cheeses are dietary staples. At the time, my mother only knew that a man who slept beneath a picture of his dog and kept hams and cheeses by his bedside possessed an innocent charm.

Four years and many prosciutto and provolone sandwiches later—in the spring of 1963—my parents were married. A year later, I was born.

⁘

LOOKING BACK, MY childhood was one big banquet. Almost every Saturday night, my parents threw dinner parties, get-out-the-wedding-silver events that allowed my father to indulge in trying new recipes, his favorite way to unwind after a stressful week working as a Madison Avenue advertising executive. My mom, a highly social creature, loved having an excuse to invite her friends over. Many Saturday mornings, I'd wake up and pad down the hall to my parents' room where I'd find Dad sitting cross-legged on the bed, surrounded by open cookbooks.

One morning he was busy studying Marcella Hazan's *The Classic Italian Cook Book*. Hazan is credited with changing America's clichéd notion of Italian food. Italian cooking, she instructed, is not overcooked spaghetti drowned in a pool of red sauce, but rather a cuisine that varies greatly from region to region, yet is bound together by a reliance on fresh, local ingredients and simple preparation.

Dad was smoking a cigarette and scribbling down a list of needed ingredients.

"Morning, sweetheart," he said. "How does *bucatini all'Amatriciana* sound to you? We'll have to make a stop at Russo's to get some pancetta."

Every Saturday after breakfast, Dad and I would drive all over western Long Island, looking for hard-to-find ingredients: saffron for *paella Valenciana*, garlic sausage for Alsatian *charcroute*, or phyllo dough for Greek *spanakopita*. In addition to Julia Child's *Mastering the Art of French Cooking* and Craig Claiborne's *The New York Times International Cook Book*, Dad was delving into Diana Kennedy's *The Cuisines of Mexico* and Madhur Jaffrey's *An Invitation to Indian Cooking*, two titles at the forefront of America's growing interest in authentic ethnic cooking.

During those dinner parties, I'd sneak downstairs just so I could peer into the dining room. The chandelier lights would be dimmed, bathing the diners in a halo of warm light. If it were winter, Dad might have prepared a hearty menu to stamp out the chill—for instance, *osso buco*, regal veal shanks resting on a golden throne of risotto Milanese with cremini mushrooms. I'd watch the blue-eye-shadowed and sideburned couples at work on their plates, their eyes glazing over. "Good God, Gary, where did you learn to cook like this?" his friend Bob would exclaim.

"Gary taught himself to cook," Mom would respond proudly.

Mom's friend Pat would turn to her and whisper, "Do you have any idea how lucky you are? My Lester can't even boil an egg."

At the end of the main course, mom and the other women

would clear the table and retire to the kitchen to wash dishes and make coffee. Dad would pull out decanters and pour brandy and other gold liquids. The men puffed on cigarettes and talked sports, waiting for their wives to bring in dessert. Even though Dad was more at home in the kitchen than any other Garden City father I knew, he still wasn't willing to assume the less glamorous aspects of meal preparation. He considered himself exempt from doing any of the pots or dishes and always left a huge mess. For him, cooking had become an exalted hobby, not a dull chore that included plunging his hands in dirty dishwater. On weeknights, it was Mom who hustled to get dinner on the table. She stuck to food that was nourishing and easy to prepare—pork chops with applesauce, or a big pot of split peas and ham. There simply wasn't enough time for the fancier approach my father employed on the weekends.

Dad would never have described himself as a home cook. Instead, he would have said he was a serious student of gastronomy, a devotee of Auguste Escoffier. In the 1970s, the world of professional kitchens was still dominated by men, and this was the world my father aligned himself with—not the world of Betty Crocker.

Although women have been the primary food providers since the beginning of recorded time, they have been unwelcome in professional kitchens until very recently. In 1971, the *Random House Dictionary* defined the word "chef" as "a cook, especially a male head cook." In that same year, however, a restaurant revolution was under way. Alice Waters was busy birthing California cuisine at Chez Panisse in Berkeley, California, paving the way for female chefs to gain serious recognition in the coming decades.

Ten years before Alice there was Julia, and it was mainly Julia who allowed Dad to play the role of home chef without receiving any crap from his male peers. *Mastering the Art of French Cooking*, by Julia Child, Simone Beck, and Loisette Berthole, published in 1961, inspired legions of serious home cooks. Appearing that same year was *The New York Times Cook Book*, written by Craig Claiborne, the paper's high-profile restaurant critic and food editor. Both books had enormous influence, making haute cuisine accessible to the American home cook. The vast majority of these gourmets-in-training were homemakers of the female persuasion. Yet, because these cookbooks introduced Americans to food they had previously only experienced in restaurants—extraordinary cuisine as opposed to ordinary everyday food—home cooking could be elevated from a domestic duty to an art form. This was cooking previously reserved for the male domain of professional cooking, and thus, men could finally feel safe entering the home kitchen.

In 1965, Julia Child appeared on the cover of *Time* magazine with the cover line "Everyone's in the Kitchen." The article included captioned photographs of Vice President Hubert Humphrey and August Busch III of Anheuser-Busch, among other men, all busy chopping, dicing, and stirring in their home kitchens.

Whether he was aware of it or not, by whipping up *boeuf bourguignon* as opposed to Hamburger Helper, Dad kept his masculinity intact.

⁘

IN 1986, WHEN I met my future husband, Randy, at school in Boulder, he was a culinary neophyte with a tumble of curly dark hair and deep-set blue eyes. He came from Greeley, Colorado, home of one of the largest cattle feed lots in the world—true meat-and-potatoes country. Luckily, he was ready and willing to experiment. I fed him tangles of fresh pasta held together with melted Brie and garnished with chopped tomatoes and strands of fresh basil, as well as pencil-thin asparagus wrapped in prosciutto, favorites of mine from *The Silver Palate Cookbook*. Created by successful New York City caterers Julee Rosso and Sheila Lukins, Silver Palate recipes oozed with '80s excess—from new potatoes with black caviar to twice-baked potatoes stuffed with lobster.

After graduation, I packed up my Cuisinart and headed east with Randy. We settled into a one-bedroom apartment with a tiny kitchen on Manhattan's Upper West Side. No longer supported by my parents, I had to reduce my recipe repertoire to budget-conscious items like brown rice and steamed vegetables. It didn't matter. The excitement of new love made up for the temporary blandness in our diets. Our biggest indulgence was having friends over for weekend brunch, the one meal Randy always prepared. In college, Randy did time as a dishwasher in a large chain restaurant specializing in greasy griddle items. When Randy hit a home run for the restaurant's baseball team, the manager promoted him to line cook. On the line, Randy worked under the tutelage of an ex-army cook who taught him the fine art of short-order cooking. On those weekend mornings in NYC, I'd sip Bloody Marys with our friends as Randy whipped up perfectly folded omelets, crisp hash browns, and tall stacks of buttermilk pancakes—pure comfort food that nourished the hangovers we'd acquired after bar-hopping in the East Village the night before.

The ritual of Sunday dinner at my grandparents ended with the death of Grandfather. We began eating with my parents, who had traded their suburban home for an apartment on the Upper East Side, a cross-town bus trip away. One Sunday afternoon Randy joined Dad on his traditional grocery ride. He told me later their journey began on the Upper West Side at Citarella, where they purchased jumbo shrimp, then they sped downtown to the Sullivan Street Bakery in SoHo for semolina bread, the East Village cheese shop for Gorgonzola and Asiago, and Veniero's for cannolis and other Italian pastries. In between, they checked four different gourmet groceries looking for fennel, but alas, turned up empty-handed.

Dad marched through the front door with a grim expression. "We'll have to settle for spinach risotto," he said.

Randy followed in line behind him, saddled with all the grocery bags. "I think your dad is completely nuts," he whispered.

"Randy, my boy, help me peel the shrimp," Dad called from the kitchen.

Over the years, Dad had become more and more authoritarian in the kitchen. Not surprisingly, his power trip as a chef coincided with his rise to CEO at the ad agency. At home, he behaved as executive chef, recruiting whoever was on hand to wash baby lettuces, julienne beets, shell peas, and, of course, do all the dishes. It was the late 1980s, and more and more chefs were moving into the realm of celebrity. Dad believed he had attained star status like Cajun king Paul Prudhomme, trendy pizza guru Wolfgang Puck, and ultra stylist Martha Stewart, to name a few of the decade's heavy hitters. He needed to be pampered with support staff. We didn't mind indulging him as long as we could enjoy the meals he put forth.

⁘

IN 1993 MY father was diagnosed with lung cancer. He was fifty-three years old. As the disease rapidly progressed, the feasting at home came to an end. When Dad started to lose weight, my mother, my sister Rosemary, Randy, and I ran to the kitchen to make his favorite foods. Night after night, we brought trays weighed down with rich, caloric dishes to his bedside: meatloaf and mashed potatoes, fettuccine Alfredo, and chocolate mousse. But the food went untouched. The man who had woken up every morning of his adult life and mapped out what he was going to eat that day had been robbed of his appetite.

The cancer altered Dad's well-fed appearance, too. His swarthy Mediterranean skin became sallow and gray, his cheeks hollowed, his ribs protruded. Eight weeks after the diagnosis, he was dead.

I stopped cooking. Randy and I began ordering takeout from mediocre Chinese restaurants and pizza places. It was impossible to enjoy food without thinking of Dad.

Then at the end of that first year of mourning, my mother decided to host a barbecue at her summerhouse on Long Island. She invited thirty people and asked Randy and me to pitch in.

"Randy, do you think you can grill this?" Mom asked, tossing him a couple hundred dollars worth of beef tenderloin.

He gulped. "No problem."

I volunteered to make cheese puffs, a foolproof appetizer handed down from my paternal grandmother, Marge. I was too intimidated to try something more ambitious. The friends my mother had invited over were all accustomed to Dad's flawless cooking.

That night, as Randy nervously manned the grill, a family friend named Tom swung his arm over Randy's shoulder. "Um, I think you better put the grill cover on if you want the meat to be ready before midnight," he advised, realizing Randy was in over his head. Dad must have been looking down on us because the meat turned out perfectly medium rare, and the guests raved.

A change occurred in Randy after that night. Perhaps it was the buzz he experienced from the adulation of the dinner guests. Or maybe it was the pressure to fill Dad's shoes. But Randy began tuning into Food Network, the cable-television network launched in November 1993—four months after Dad's death—that now reaches over 71 million households. Mario Batali showed Randy how to make risotto; Susan Feniger and Mary Sue Milliken, the Too Hot Tamales, taught him about mole; hunky Bobby Flay introduced him to dry rubs; and that boisterous Emeril Lagasse told him not to be afraid to "kick it up a notch" with bold seasonings. Before long, Randy was making polenta triangles topped with wild mushrooms; grilled tuna steaks marinated in ginger, lime, and soy; and rock shrimp quesadillas topped with mango salsa. On Saturday nights, we began to throw serious dinner parties. We got into the habit of running all over the city, searching for the best ingredients: the Union Square Greenmarket for the freshest produce, Florence Meat Market for the best steaks, the Gourmet Garage for great olives.

After the parties we kick off our shoes and pour each other a glass of port. Then we take turns washing and drying the dishes.

Randy has evolved into a "foodie," though no one seems to find Randy's interest in cooking that unusual. Today, a man hunkered down over a cutting board in the kitchen isn't such a rarity as it was when my dad first started cooking. As we begin the twenty-first century, men seem as comfortable in the home kitchen as women have become in professional kitchens.

⸙

RANDY AND I have a three-year-old son, Gary, whom we named after my father. On Saturday mornings Gary runs into our bedroom and tugs Randy's arm.

"Dad, it's time to make pancakes," he says. Then he turns to me. "You stay here, Mom."

I sink back under the covers as the men head to the kitchen.

gary's risotto milanese with cremini mushrooms

1 cup dry white wine
1 lb. cremini mushrooms
4 T. olive oil
¾ cup chopped yellow onion
2 cups Arborio rice
6–7 cups chicken or beef broth (if you use canned,
mix 1 can of water with every 2 cans of broth)
¼ tsp. saffron threads dissolved in a few teaspoons of hot water
1 cup grated Parmesan cheese
salt and pepper to taste

In a sauté pan, sauté mushrooms in one tablespoon of olive oil for five minutes, until mushrooms render their juices. Set aside. In another heavy pot, sauté onion in remaining olive oil over medium flame. Meanwhile, bring broth to boil in a saucepan, reduce heat, and keep at a lively simmer. When onion is soft, add rice and cook another three minutes until rice is translucent. Slowly add the wine to the rice and stir occasionally until the liquid has been absorbed, then add a cup of broth, stir, and simmer until the liquid is absorbed. Add the mushrooms and their juices, the saffron, and about half a cup of broth, stirring constantly until the liquid is absorbed. Add the remaining broth about a half-cup at a time, stirring until the rice is slightly creamy, tender but firm to the bite (about twenty minutes total cooking time). Remove from heat. Stir in Parmesan cheese, salt, and pepper to taste. Serve immediately with extra grated Parmesan.

food before sanity

{ L E L A   N A R G I }

I RECENTLY FIRED my therapist. Actually, to be honest, in the last eight months I have fired two therapists. I fired the first one after she recommended a novel to me—her "new favorite," she said—that was so trite, so poorly written, that, as much as it pained me, I had to admit I'd lost all respect for her. Call this firing a simple case of literary snobbery, then. As for the second therapist, I fired her for a slightly more complicated reason. I fired her because she insisted on talking about food.

I should explain first of all that I am not overweight. I am not now, nor have I ever been, anorexic, bulimic, or even anemic. I never thought of myself as a person with "food issues." Look at my childhood, an idyll of cookery. An average day found my mother in the kitchen, flitting from fridge to stove to cabinets. With great competence and no small amount of panache, she could stir the contents of a pot, shake a skillet, season something freshly ladled from the pressure cooker, toss a salad, and remove two loaves of bread to cool on a wire rack with hands padded by lobster-like oven mitts. On my birthday, she would decorate a three-tiered cake with elaborate piping and lavender-icing flowers she spent a whole day coaxing through a decorator's tube, petal by petal. On other special occasions, she let me thumb through her cookbooks and pick the menu. My favorite was the Japanese cookbook, a folio of large cards with recipes in both English and Japanese on one side, photos of the finished dish on the other. In the photos all the food looked like treasure: Carrots were carved like swans, slices of fish were rolled like roses, grains of rice gleamed like seed pearls. "Food is magic," the book seemed to whisper. And I believed it.

I believe it even now. Every summer Saturday finds me at the farmers' market, gasping in disbelief at the sights and smells of over-abundance. How to choose from forty varieties of lettuce; how could there *be* forty varieties of lettuce? The intoxicating scent of peaches is so potent that I can follow it, past the fragrant melons and the explosively sweet-smelling cherries, all the way to the stall at the far end of the market.

Then there is the taste of a truly fresh egg, subtle and buttery. It is my gladdening companion through a forty-five-minute wait on a farm-stand line. Other marketers pass as I wait along with sixty or more like-minded egg lovers.

"Wow, look at this line," the passersby marvel. "What are you all waiting for?"

"Eggs," we say, smirking, waiting for the unvarying response of: *"Eggs!"* A shake of the head, a bemused frown, a muttering to a companion as the disbeliever wanders away from the line: "They're waiting for *eggs!*"

Of course what the disbelievers do not know, what everyone waiting on line *does* know, is that we are not really waiting for eggs. We are waiting for a vessel of suspended disbelief: a taste that will satisfy beyond our wildest imaginings, make us catch our breath, then groan in amazement; a vehicle that will transport us beyond the world of "eggs" and into the far superior kingdom of "Eggs!" A tomato can be such a vessel, too; so can a chocolate cake. This is why food is magic. It holds infinite, unprecedented delights, never exhausted.

People don't believe that I eat much. I am skinny, have lived my whole life as a skinny person. Consequently, I have lived with scorn. People don't seem to hold much stock in the positive powers of genetics. My mother is skinny, so was my father, so are all my cousins and grandparents. People don't consider this proof. I can almost hear their brains grinding over meatier possibilities: a family of bulimics, a family addicted to painkillers, a whole family infected with a rare stomach disease. Sometimes I let people off the hook with a lie, tell them we are a family of alcoholic chain-smokers, and watch as their faces are consumed by relief.

Nor do people believe me when I say that I don't really care much for junk food. They test me: French fries? Potato chips? Cheez Doodles? Doritos? Hostess cupcakes? Mallomars? M&M's? Listen, I tell them, I'm a person who will follow my nose three blocks to get at a bushel of peaches. Candy, snack foods, they hardly rate by comparison. I've been this way since I was a girl; at the age of seven I braved cafeteria taunts in order to eat niçoise olives and my beloved lupini beans with lunch. I knew nothing then about junk food. This was because my mother shunned Snickers in favor of figs and homemade peanut butter; her pots and pans were never disgraced by the addition of packaged mac and cheese, or canned ravioli.

Having brought up my mother for the third time now, maybe I should draw this excursus back around to where I began, with my therapist. My therapist, naturally, was always keen to link my every motive, my every small utterance to my mother. Our last conversation, two days before I left her a cowardly phone message explaining that we were through for good, was no exception. A reenactment:

SHE: Let's talk about food today.

ME   (*Puzzled*): Um, okay.

SHE: How do you feel about food?

ME: How do I feel about food? What do you mean?

SHE: Do you like food? Do you hate food? Are you ambivalent about food? *What does food mean to you?*

ME: Uh, I guess you could say I love food. I love to cook. I love to eat . . .

SHE: Interesting. . . . What do you love to eat?

ME: Gee, I don't know. All kinds of things.

SHE: You must be more specific.

Let me interrupt this scintillating dialogue for a moment to explain that by the time this conversation is taking place I have already been suspecting, for a number of weeks, that my therapist is not a food-lover. She barely batted an eyelash on my first visit, when I told her I'd published a cookbook; a food-lover, even a professionally disengaged psychotherapist food-lover, would want to know more. In her office, a faint aroma of garlic, or apples, or any giveaway as to what was ingested for lunch, never lingers. Therapists eat at their desks—quickly, granted, but you'd think some lunch smell would stick—and the chronic, unvarying scent of carpet and hot light bulbs in my therapist's office makes me think perhaps she does not even like the smell of food. Finally, my hunch: she just doesn't look like the kind of person who cooks. I can't imagine her juggling spices, or grease-splattering her kitchen. She is definitely takeout material. What do you tell a person like this when they ask you what you like to eat, especially when you're the kind of person who waits forty-five minutes in line to buy fresh eggs?

ME: I like just about everything, any good food. I can't pick favorites.

SHE: What *don't* you like to eat?

ME: Turnips. Oh, and I don't like cooked peppers mixed into a dish, although on their own they're fine. And I'm not overly fond of the taste of bergamot.

SHE (*Looking exasperated but determined not to ask me what bergamot is*): "Let's try this another way. What do you normally eat for breakfast?"

ME: Well, except on weekends I don't spend a lot of time on breakfast. Usually, I just eat toast, or a banana. I like to eat quickly so I can get to my desk and start writing.

SHE (*Looking delighted, like she might actually utter the word "Aha!"*): Ahhhh . . . so you hate to eat breakfast.

To interject again: how do you explain to someone who is not a food-lover that if you are the kind of person who likes all flavors except turnip and bergamot, you might also be the kind of person who really enjoys a plain banana when it is perfectly ripe, with a firm texture and no brown spots; that, in fact, you can hardly imagine a better breakfast because this one really does it for you, really satisfies?

ME (*Trapped into virtual non sequitur*): Actually, I love bananas.

SHE: But you don't like toast. . . .

ME: [*Confused silence*]

SHE: What about your childhood? Did your mother cook?

ME: My mother was a fabulous cook. She made gourmet, five-course dinners every night, and that was in addition to going to work, taking care of me, doing all the shopping, and cleaning up.

SHE: And your father did *nothing?*

ME: That's right.

SHE: Did your mother actually *like* to cook?

ME: Well, yes. My father may have been a domineering jerk who never lifted a finger around the house, but he never forced my mother to make *bouillabaisse*, or Peking duck, or *coq au vin*. He would have eaten any swill she served up. She cooked these things because she liked to cook them.

SHE: Hmmm. And now you like to cook. That's interesting. How did you feel as a girl when your mother would make these elaborate meals? How did it make you feel about your father?

And here I will leave off the dialogue. If it wasn't bad enough that we were going to talk (again) about my mother, adding my father to the mix was really deflating my desire to "discover" anything about my relationship with food (a relationship, I learned at the end of our session, my therapist had been convinced was based on anorexia, since I'm so skinny). Because what does the above conversation really conjure? An unhappy American family circa 1973, with a father who does no housework, a mother who does all the cooking, two parents who still accept—it is 1973 after all, the year almost no one imagined Billie Jean King could trounce flabby Bobby Riggs in a so-called Battle of the Sexes—that in most American households this is normal. (Of course, it was somewhat less normal in 1978, when my mother finally left my father, thereby joining the legions of divorced single mothers who no longer had the time or the stamina to prepare five-course dinners.) Really, there is only one circumstance in this brief plunge into my childhood that someone might consider slightly out-of-the-ordinary, and that is that my mother was a mighty and accomplished cook.

People who do not cook are suspicious of this talent in others.

I learned to cook from my mother. When I say "learned," I don't mean that she gave me lessons, or even that I spent much time watching her in the kitchen. I learned to cook by recognizing my mother's love for food. This I learned through osmosis, as I learned to react to an annoying bit of news by watching how my mother tightened her lips slightly and let her eyes go blank. And as I learned to be afraid to sing in public, because she is. Daughters learn plenty of things from their mothers without even wanting to. Not all these things are stimulating fodder worthy of the cost of a visit to the psychotherapist's office.

My mother's love of food was palpable, inspiring. She would hunker down with her cookbooks, giving them a good going-over every now and again as if she were re-reading a favorite novel. She liked to pick up strange foodstuffs in the supermarket, to experiment with: In 1973, dried poblano peppers were exotic; so was eel. Her eyes would take on a confident, conquering spark when she contemplated the tidy rows of fruits and vegetables at the greengrocer's, coming to rest on the plumpest, the most inevitably delicious.

My mother was all concentration when she cooked; nothing could distract her. She wore in the kitchen an expression of intense calm. Not every new dish was a triumph, but she never second-guessed herself, never lost confidence. The kitchen is the only place where I've seen her approach joy. In the kitchen she was completely absorbed, absolutely herself. These things I say about my mother— most of them, now, also apply to me. Like my mother, I love food and all things related to it.

I fired my therapist because she didn't love food. I suppose you could say this was petty. But a person who does not love food cannot understand this propensity in others, cannot feel empathy for their disposition. They do not realize that, for a food-lover, to draw food into the realm of "issues" and family is to ruin its magic forever. By the age of twenty, all daughters know they are like their mothers, and all daughters wish they were less so. By the age of thirty, most daughters are exhausted by the prospect of another ten years of battling the onslaught of motherlike tendencies. With a sigh, we resign ourselves to any number of cringe-worthy similarities. Positive associations we admit quietly.

I learned to love food through my mother, maybe even—to throw a bone to therapists—in spite of my mother. Purely within the context of eating and food, it does not matter to me that my father never did the grocery shopping. Or that my mother, perhaps, used elaborate cookery as a way to gain some distance, as a way to remove herself for hours at a time from the daily drudgery of her wifely and motherly existence.

From my mother, too, I learned to love cooking. I do not want to question why I love to cook. Would it really matter if I did so in order to gain my mother's approval? Or because I had some deep-seated need to take care of people? Or to satisfy my ego? To love food, and to love to cook—why should I want to analyze these loves away?

Some evenings at dinnertime, I catch myself flitting around my own kitchen in mindful oblivion, and recognize my mother in action. I take a brief moment to settle into this concordance, standing there amid the cheerful detritus of another night's cooking experiment—spills of saffron and cumin, a few dirty spoons, stovetop splatters of every shape and color—and imagine how my ex-therapist would balk at the scene.

SHE: You mean to tell me that you just let the sauce *bubble over* like that, all over the kitchen, and didn't even clean it up?

ME: Yes. Then, after I ate my meal straight out of the pot, I let the dog lick sauce off my chin. She's always been a big fan of my cooking.

fundamental pleasures

{ AMANDA HESSER }

I LEFT THE paper at ten of eight, walking out into the aggressive neon of Times Square, loaded down with a shopping bag filled with papers, a cookbook, and a bottle of olive oil. My eyes felt shrunken from the office's fluorescent lighting, from squinting at my computer screen. I dipped into the subway station. A scattering of people stood on the platform looking down the tunnel, down at their papers, anywhere but at each other.

I wondered, as I often do: What will they eat when they get home? For the middle-aged man with the beat-up briefcase, will it be a cold slab of lasagna, pulled from the refrigerator and eaten while standing, his fork pawing at the food? Will the woman in clunky shoes be greeted with a steaming lamb curry prepared by her husband? Or will her meal be a glass of cheap wine and a morsel of cheese, consumed on the sofa in front of the TV?

I didn't know exactly what I would be having for dinner, but I knew what I needed. My husband was away on business, and I knew our apartment would feel dead without him, so I needed to put a pan on the stove and feel heat lapping up its sides. I needed to feel the scratch of salt between my fingertips as I sprinkled it over my food. I needed my placemat on the table, the Japanese lantern above the table lit and low, the trickle of wine being poured slowly into a glass.

I buried my head in a book and waited for the subway to careen under the East River to my stop just on the other side, in Brooklyn. Peas & Pickles, a local grocery, was empty. The man at the cash register was taking strawberries out of large flats and arranging them in small cartons, putting the largest ones on top. I picked up a dozen eggs, a persimmon, a bunch of thin leeks and some tarragon, and headed home, assembling the ingredients in my mental kitchen. I'd poach the egg, I thought, and melt, as the French say, the leeks in butter with a pinch of tarragon. That would be plenty.

When someone first learns to cook, some of the most basic skills—poaching an egg, sautéing a fillet of fish, and boiling pasta— can seem daunting, even infuriating. So much effort for such plain food. It can feel like it will take years to learn to compose "real" cuisine with its layering of flavors, herb oils, and reduced sauces. And it will, for most cooks at least.

And it will probably take many more—as it did for me— to realize that while preparing complex dishes and course-upon-course dinner parties is a splendid accomplishment, some of the most pleasing dishes emerge from the early stages of one's culinary life. Dressing noodles with freshly grated nutmeg, butter, and Parmesan cheese. Rolling asparagus in frothy butter. Roasting small potatoes until they caramelize on the edges and their skins wrinkle.

⫶

A FEW YEARS ago, I took a new writing job—my first full-time job—and was quickly swept up in long wearying days at work. I was living in a new city with few friends and little time for the ones I had. I fought staggering waves of loneliness like I had never experienced, and when they hit I began to crave eggs and toast, orange slices and tea, the foods that my mother fed to me when I was sick. I might wilt spinach in butter and olive oil, slice romaine for a chopped salad, mash butternut squash with a little crème fraiche. Dessert was often ice cream and a cognac.

I trudged through cooking. It seemed so chore-like when the results were so mundane. Yet repetition became a powerful source of comfort. While my schedule stayed the same (maybe I even liked it, latched on to my busy-ness as a source of pride), with time—age—I changed. I wanted to slow things down elsewhere. And in the kitchen, I could. I grew to like pounding my fist on the blade of my knife to split open a clove of garlic. I enjoyed watching a piece of fish shrink at the edges in the heat of the oven. I no longer minded whisking mustard and vinegar for a vinaigrette. The meals were sound; I could recall the flavors, and began to enjoy not having worked too hard to feed myself well. I knew what I was doing, and the results had the purity and consolation of childhood memories.

I once read that M.F.K. Fisher would sometimes have fruit and a glass of cold milk for lunch. At the time, this struck me as austere, a puzzling ritual in a life lived so richly. Around that time, I visited a friend who was a chef. As we talked, she made herself a little lunch before going to work. She pulled a sweet potato out of her toaster oven, split it open and sprinkled sea salt inside. She did this with great care, then ate it slowly. Now, I understand what both women were up to.

This is a cuisine for which there are few recipes. While it is no longer acceptable to include a recipe for poaching eggs in a cookbook (unless a salsa verde or olive oil sabayon follows), everyone knows that a poached egg with a dash of salt is a combination that cannot be improved upon. The exterior of the egg sheets in the simmering water. Inside, the whites are like velvety curd and the yolk becomes its luxurious sauce. Such delectables are the great secrets of the kitchen, a testament to fundamental pleasures.

Edouard de Pomiane did his best to capture such plain treats in *Cooking with Pomiane*: "For a gourmand there is no need to produce complicated dishes with fancy names," he wrote. "Prepare for him raw materials of good quality. Transform them as little as possible and accompany them with suitable sauces and you will have produced a meal which is just right."

His pumpkin soup is cooked in a single pot and contains merely pumpkin, milk, and rice. He gives instructions for *croutes au fromage*, or grilled cheeses, and includes how and when to serve chilled white wine with them. Chives on toast are precisely that, creamed with butter and a "dusting of pepper."

Eating well, de Pomiane believed, made you a whole and "normal" person. Those who did not were likely to be "unhappy, embittered, pessimistic, disagreeable, and even dangerous." I can agree with the first part—eating well does help replenish the mind and improve one's outlook, even if it is only a post-meal high, which then fades like a sunset. The act of preparing yourself a meal is edifying, as well. Your hands, having left the computer keyboard or steering wheel, are put to use with their much more primal function, as tools. You must use your senses. And while many daily projects are left with loose ends, a meal is not. It has a beginning, middle, and end.

De Pomiane died in 1964. He would probably be frustrated by the current polarization of American cooks into those who do not have time to cook and those who love cooking so much that they can't stop themselves from pursuing the latest culinary obsessions. He would want to tidy up our kitchens and set us back on course.

But we can still turn back to him, and to his delight in carrots with cream and pork chops with rhubarb. Or we can find our own way. Occasionally, now, I will have fruit and milky coffee for lunch. Or toast with butter and jam. A piece of creamy cheese.

❖

AFTER SHOPPING THAT evening on my way home from work, I arrived home to an empty apartment. I flicked on the kitchen light, cleared the counter, and pulled out my large knife and sauté pan. I poured myself a glass of sherry. There were no recipes to turn to. I simply knew that to soften leeks, you must cook them slowly in a thin coating of fat. There was no need for a timer. I would stand over them and watch the chemistry take place. I would drop in a little chopped tarragon at the end, then taste a spoonful to see. Rinsing the leeks, spreading the firm layers under the faucet, was the first order of business. I sliced them in half and leaned into the sink, letting the ropey stream of warm water run over my hands.

school lunch

{ POOJA MAKHIJANI }

Mom says she is being "sensible" about what I eat and she likes to pack "sensible" lunches. Plastic sandwich bags filled with blood-red pomegranate seeds. Fresh raisin bread wrapped in foil. Homemade vegetable biryani made with brown rice and lima beans. Yellow pressed rice with potatoes and onions. A silver thermos full of warm tamarind-infused lentil soup. Blue and white Tupperware containers that can be reused. Lunch sacks that have to be brought home every day. Silverware.

I don't want her lunches. I want to touch a cold, red Coca-Cola can that will hiss when I open it. I want to pull out a yellow Lunchables box so I can assemble bite-size sandwiches with Ritz crackers and smoked turkey. I want to smell tuna salad with mayonnaise and pickles. I want bologna on white bread, Capri Sun Fruit Punch, and Cool Ranch Doritos in a brown paper bag. I want plastic forks that I can throw away when I am done eating. But I am too scared to ask her. I know she will say, "No."

❖

"WHY DON'T YOU invite Chrissy over this Friday after school?" Mom ladles a spoonful of sweetened, homemade yogurt into a white ceramic bowl. "You've already been to her house twice." I hoist myself onto one of the high chairs at my kitchen table and pull my breakfast toward me. I tear the hot masala roti into eight irregular pieces and dip the largest one into the cold yogurt.

"I will, I will." I rub my fingers on the paper towel in my lap. The last time I went to Chrissy's house, Mrs. Pizarro gave us mini–hot dogs wrapped in pastry topped with a squirt of mustard, and tall glasses of Hawaiian Punch as an after-school snack. I can't imagine Chrissy coming to our house and munching on cauliflower and broccoli florets while gulping down chilled milk. I don't want to think about all the questions she will ask: When she sees the bronze Ganesh idol on the wooden stool near the sofa, she will inquire, *What is that elephant-headed statue in your living room?* When she sniffs the odor of spices that permeates the bedrooms, she will question, *What's the smell?* And when she accidentally touches my mother's henna colored sari, she will query, *What's your mom wearing?*

"I will," I say between bites so Mom won't ask me again. "Just not this week."

She glances at the clock on the oven. "Hurry up with your food, beti. Nishaat Aunty will be here any second." She grabs the rest of the roti, dunks it into the yogurt. and shovels it into my mouth. Thick globs of yogurt slide in rivulets down her palms and she licks it off once I am done eating. She wipes her hands on her red gingham apron and hands me a bulging brown paper bag. "Your lunch," she says.

"What did you pack today?" I ask as I shove the bag into my purple canvas backpack alongside my spelling and math textbooks.

"Aloo tikkis. Left over from last night."

"Oh." I part the curtains of the kitchen window and look for Nishaat Aunty's midnight-blue station wagon. "Chrissy brought Coke with her to school yesterday." I look into her eyes, hoping she will understand.

"Coca-Cola! During school?" she says. "Of course, that's what those American parents do. That's why their children are so hyper and don't concentrate on their studies." I am not allowed to drink soda, except on Saturdays when Mom makes fried fish. Recently, I've been drinking lots of apple juice because she is worried that there is too much acidity in orange juice.

⁖

"OKAY, CLASS, TIME for lunch." Miss Brown, my fifth-grade teacher, puts down the piece of chalk and rubs her hands on her chocolate-brown pleated pants, leaving behind ghostly prints. She grabs her cardigan off her chair and heads to the teachers' lounge near the gym.

Our lunch aide, Ms. Bauer, walks into the classroom. Her long silver hair cascades over her shoulders and down her back, hiding her ears.

"Row One, you can go to the closets and get your money or your food," Ms. Bauer's raspy voice instructs the five students in the front of the room. I wait for her to call "Row Four" so I can run to the back of the classroom and yank my sack off the top shelf of the closet. Every day, I take my food out of my sack and slide it into my desk. I leave it there until the end of the day so I can throw it away in the large garbage bin next to Principal Ward's office before I head for home.

"Row Two." I look out the window. I see the rusty swing set in the front of Washington School. Before Christmas, there were three wooden planks attached to the bar. This spring, only one remains and it sways, lonely, in an early April breeze.

"Row Three." By now, several of my classmates have lined up near the globes in front of the room. They will wait there until everyone whose parents gave them a dollar and two quarters this morning have lined up. Ms. Bauer will walk them down the hall to the temporary lunch stations and they will bring back compartmentalized Styrofoam trays loaded with food.

"Row Four." I bolt. As I reach for my sack, I feel someone tug on my pink turtleneck. I turn around to see who tapped me on the shoulder.

"Aisha." She reintroduces herself.

It's the new girl. Mr. Ward brought her to our classroom on Monday, right after we had finished the Pledge of Allegiance. "Aisha's family just came from Pakistan two days ago," he said. "Please make her feel welcome."

Miss Brown rearranged our desks a bit, and put Aisha in the center of the room. Then she pulled down the world map and gave everyone a quick geography lesson. "Now, who can find Pakistan?" she asked. Even though I knew, I didn't raise my hand. Months before, we'd studied India and Pakistan and Bangladesh in our South Asia unit in social studies. As we took turns reading aloud paragraphs, Miss Brown asked me to read the longest section on the topography of the subcontinent. "And in the northeast, Nepal is separated from Tibet by the mighty Himalayan Mountains." I concluded as I heard snickers behind me.

"Hima-aaa-layan," Eddie whispered to no one in particular.

"It's Him-a-lay-an." Miss Brown corrected me at the same time. An accent on the first syllable. Short 'a' sounds. Four quick strokes and not the drawn-out vowels that had rolled off my tongue.

I wasn't going to pronounce "Pakistan" the way I knew how to— with a hissing "st" sound not heard in the English language.

"Will you have lunch at my desk today?" she asks. Today, just like yesterday, she wears her fanciest salwaar khameez to school. Yesterday, she wore a blue kurta over a satin white churidaar, and today she wears a shimmery lavender top decorated with clusters of pearls along the edges. She slings her dupatta over her left shoulder. It is longer in the front than in the back and the end gets caught in the heel of her white chappal.

I look down at my cuffed jeans and wonder if she wants to wear sneakers. Will everyone ask Aisha questions about what she is wearing, why she has an accent, or where she comes from? I have always said "No, thank you" when Chrissy or Heather have asked me to eat with them because I don't want to explain anything that makes me different from them. Will I have to explain things about Aisha too? I don't know whether to say yes and be nice, or say no, and read a book while waiting for recess.

"Sure, I'll eat with you," I say finally. I know she has asked me to sit at her desk because I am the only person in the classroom who looks somewhat like her.

She looks relieved. "I have to go buy some food." She rummages through her fleece-lined jacket and takes out $1.50. "Pull your chair up to my desk. I will be back in ten minutes." I watch her get into the lunch line that Ms. Bauer directs out the door.

I drag my chair over to the front of the room. I haven't had a chance to stuff my lunch into my desk, so I peer inside my bag.

I see Mom's aloo tikkis. She's stuffed the leftover potato patties inside a hard roll from La Bonbonniere bakery. The deep-fried flattened ball of potato is spiked with garam masala and shoved into a bun slathered with fresh coriander chutney, which Mom makes with coarsely ground almonds that crunch in my mouth when I least expect it. Below the sandwich are a bunch of grapes in a Ziploc bag. No dripping-wet can of Sprite. No Little Debbie apple pie. No Hostess chocolate cupcakes filled with vanilla cream. No strawberry Pop-Tarts.

I zip up my bag again and wait for Aisha to return. She brings back her tray and places it on her desk. Today's lunch is six chicken nuggets, a spoonful of corn, sticky peach halves floating in sugar syrup, and a tough dinner roll.

"I thought you would have started eating by now." Aisha pierces her chocolate milk carton with a straw.

"I am not that hungry." My stomach growls. I am used to ignoring the sounds. I can usually get through the day on the normal, easily-explainable-if-anyone-sees food. Carrot sticks, apple slices, or Saltines.

"But you brought your lunch. I saw you take something out of that bag. What is it?" she insists.

I reach inside my bag and feel the crusty bread. I draw it out, pressing it between my fingers and thumb, flattening it into a tiny Frisbee, mashing the roll into the soft potatoes.

"See, it is just bread." The disk is so flat that you can't see the tikki inside.

"No, there's something inside it." Aisha peers at the sandwich. "Is that an aloo tikki in a bun? I wish my mother would pack them in my lunch for me. Yesterday, I bought peanut-butter-and-jelly sandwiches. I've never had peanut butter before. It's such a funny food. It stuck to the back of my teeth and I could taste it for the rest of the day."

I look at the flattened mess in my hands and think about licking peanut butter from the crevices in my mouth. I gaze at Aisha's chicken nuggets.

"Wanna trade?" I ask.

"Are you sure? If I were you, I'd keep my food." She cocks her head and her eyes dart between the multicolored array in front of her and the earth-tone concoction just a few inches away from her.

"If you want it, you can have it." My fingers inch over to her side of the desk.

"You can have everything except the corn. I like that." She passes her plate to me and I hand my lunch to her.

"How long have you been here?" I devour all the chicken nuggets before Aisha changes her mind.

"We just got here last weekend. We are living in Edison Village, right near the train station." She nibbles her way around the entire circumference of the bun. "You've probably been here longer than that. You sound like an American."

I realize she is commenting on the way I pronounce words. Her accent sounds like my mother's. "I was born in New York. I've lived in Edison as long as I can remember."

"Then why don't you eat the school lunch?" Aisha spoons the corn into her mouth.

I don't have an answer for Aisha. I know it's not because it's too expensive or that Styrofoam trays are environmentally unsound. It's because Mom thinks her deep-fried aloo tikkis and freshly ground masalas are what good Indian parents give their daughters. She doesn't understand that good Indian daughters just want to become American.

It's too complicated an issue to explain. Like my mother, Aisha won't understand it.

"Time for recess." Ms. Bauer claps her hands three times. I throw the tray and the plastic utensils in the garbage can in the front of the room, and Aisha walks with me back to the closets to put my lunch sack back on the shelf. I race back towards the front of the line that is heading out the door, a few steps behind Chrissy and Heather, following them to the asphalt playground. The boys bolt off to play kickball, their four bases taking up most of the space on the grounds. The girls congregate near the fence around Ms. Bauer as she pulls multicolored jump ropes out of her tote bags.

"Cookies, candies in a dish. How many pieces do you wish?"

Chrissy and Heather both jump into the twirling rope. "One, two, three, four," twenty-five girls chant. "Twelve, thirteen . . ." The rope gets caught under Heather's sneaker.

"Aisha, would you like to try?" Ms. Bauer turns to Aisha and me, who both watch intently.

"Okay." She kicks off her chappals and ties her dupatta around her waist. "But I don't know any of the songs."

"Don't worry. I will pick one for you." Aisha stands between the two lunch ladies, the rope swaying in the wind against her bare feet. I collapse down onto the ground and sit, legs crossed, as I usually do, singing along, but never joining in. "Cinderella, dressed in yella. Went upstairs to see her fella. How many kisses did she get?" Aisha is jumping furiously in time with the music. "Twenty-eight, twenty-nine, thirty, thirty . . ." Aisha missteps and stumbles.

"That was fun." She sits down next to me.

I smile. "You are very good."

·❖·

"THERE IS A new girl in our class," I tell Mom after school as I peel the tangerine she's given me. "She's from Pakistan." I pull the segments apart and arrange them in a circle on the napkin.

"When did they come?"

"Last weekend." I tell her all the stories Aisha told me at lunch—about her all-girls school in Islamabad, her two younger brothers, and how busy her parents are trying to find a job in New Jersey. I pick up a single slice of the tangerine and glide it between my teeth. "She even wore Indian—I mean, Pakistani—clothes to school every day this week."

"You should do that too." She sweeps up the discarded peel with her hands.

I sink my incisors into the fruit. A burst of juice fills my mouth. "She just came from there. That's why she does it," I rationalize to her. "She doesn't have American clothes. And she eats the school lunch." I hope that she picks up on my second subtle hint of the day.

"I am sure once they are all settled in, Aisha's mother will be giving her biryani as well." She wipes the tangerine juice that's dribbled out of my mouth onto my chin, and I lower myself from the chair. "They'll want to hold onto that in this country. Don't you want your banana today?"

"No, I am not hungry. I ate lunch."

⁘

AISHA AND I continue to exchange meals for the rest of the school year. I give her more of my mom's aloo tikkis, and she hands over her pizza bagels. I demolish her macaroni and cheese, and she inhales my masala rice. Aisha starts to wear jeans by June. She always takes off her sneakers and socks before jumping rope, though; she says it's easier that way.

Every day, at 3:15, as I jump into our ice-blue Dodge Caravan, Mom asks me, "Did you finish the lunch I packed for you today?"

"Yes, Mom," I lie. I am not about to spoil my arrangement.

aloo tikki
(potato patties)

The aloo tiki is an ubiquitous Indian food and the perfect solution for leftover mashed potatoes. For an interesting variation, top them with hot chickpeas, chopped red onion, mint and coriander chutney, and golden yellow sev (thin deep-fried chickpea noodles).

5–6 medium-sized potatoes, peeled, boiled, and mashed

2 onions, finely chopped

5 cloves garlic, finely chopped

2 tsp. fresh ginger, minced

1 cup coriander leaves (cilantro), finely chopped

1 tsp. salt

1 tsp. pepper

½ tsp. cinnamon

4 T. oil

In a large bowl, mix all the ingredients and knead into a pliable dough. Divide into golf ball–sized portions and flatten into patties.

In a frying pan, heat four tablespoons of oil. Pan-fry each patty, about two minutes on each side, until golden brown.

Makes fifteen patties. Serve with ketchup or mint and coriander chutney.

mint and coriander chutney

Tamarind, mango, tomato, coconut—almost everything is transformed into a garnish in my house, but mint and coriander chutney is one of my favorites. You can hold back on the chilies if you want a milder condiment.

2 cups coriander leaves (cilantro), chopped

1 cup mint leaves, chopped

10–15 almonds

½ cup coconut, grated

4–5 green chilies

1 cup of lemon juice

1 tsp. sugar

1 T. salt

10–15 almonds, coarsely chopped (optional)

In blender, grind coriander, mint, whole almonds, coconut, chilies, lemon juice, salt, and sugar until it becomes a smooth paste. (Add water to maintain consistency.) For an extra-crunchy chutney, stir in the coarsely chopped almonds.

after birth

{ ALISA GORDANEER }

GARLIC AND ONIONS sizzling in extra-virgin olive oil weave their scent through the noon kitchen. The smell wraps around the cookware that hangs from a metal rack, glinting like the sunlight through the window on the skillets' copper bottoms. It eases past the counter piled with plates and unwashed coffee cups, and travels through the air, molecules of onion floating like specks of dust. It is breathed in through the nostrils of a woman who has recently given birth and is ravenous.

The hunger started in the hospital, after the pain and nausea subsided. The baby born, the placenta expelled into a stainless steel bowl, the breasts met by an eager, searching mouth. With the afterpains—the exhausted uterus contracting sharply with the tiny girl's every suckle—came the first fierce pangs. She embraced the hunger, answered it with salty chicken noodle soup and a plastic cup of ice cream with a wooden paddle, all the nurses could find at that dawning hour.

But the hunger continued. She listened to its pangs as the aches of labor wound their way into muscles and sinew *(afterpains, afterpains, and breathe)*. In the euphoria of that night, she felt like she was floating. Not outside life, but somehow outside herself, just floating. She focused on the hunger, the familiar nudge of body asking soul. It told her she was still connected, a tenacious but temporary hold, like the baby's mouth latched firmly to her breast. She ate one-handed, fast, the taste of vanilla and salt.

With the smell of the cooking garlic, she feels herself return, not fully to her body, but closer than she's felt for the past week. It's been that long since the pains started, regular and deep, contractions that began the separation that culminated in birth. That was the beginning of the end of things, she knows. The end of her moon-belly and the way she and her daughter were one. Now, of course, they are two. Three, counting her husband, who tends her aches with arnica and changes diapers, wrapping the squalling girl in blankets and walking, walking, walking. The nights roll into days, and days bleed into the thick gauze pads of nights. Their world tumbles into gentle tentative touches of skin and scalp and fine, fuzzed hair.

It's been a week, and her hunger has lasted, through reheated carry-out and frozen entrees tossed haphazardly into the microwave. Chicken Alfredo with some sort of noodles, hardened into a chilly block. Rice reconstituted from packets, flavored with salt and soy protein. Filling enough, between nursings and changings, naps and moments of wide-eyed, miraculous wakefulness. Filling, but not enough.

She's learned, whenever she has a free hand and a plate of food, to gobble. No longer does she linger over salad, chewing thoughtfully, carefully, swallowing with dainty sips of water. No more leisurely meals, savored bites. She ignores all flavor in the interest of fueling, stoking the fire.

Because it doesn't matter how fast or slow she consumes. No matter the creamy sauces, no matter apples sliced and eaten with caramel or bread dipped in olive oil, an hour later, she's hungry again. And the food she consumes leaks from her breasts, eagerly sucked dry by this girl she's only just met. Child of hers, made of flesh.

❖

THE SMELL IN the kitchen grows stronger as the onions caramelize, and her tongue licks her lips with carnal desire. Not lust. That's what got her here in the first place. "Carnal," from Latin *carnalis*. Flesh-eater. Meat-eater. Her carnal desire is a need for flesh. The stuff of life.

The placenta nearly filled the ice cream tub. Frozen solid, it took two days in the refrigerator to thaw, an iciness that defied the memory of how it slopped warmly from between her legs. How the midwife clamped the cord, that white, slippery rope that moored them together, and then cut the baby free and squalling. She remembers the quick, sure tug, a grunting sense of release deep inside her, and the organ plopping into the shine of a stainless steel bowl. "I want to keep that," she'd said, and someone found an empty container in the hospital's kitchen. Ice cream, vanilla, one gallon.

"Nobody's ever asked before," said the nurse. "I guess you'll plant it under a rose bush."

"No," she replied. "I'm going to eat it."

The nurse wrote something in the big black binder marked Patient Record.

❖

IN THE DAYS before the birth, when she'd had time to linger over books, she'd learned all she could about placentas. The placenta is a unique organ, she read. It does not exist unless called for, begins to grow at the moment a fertilized egg is implanted in the uterus. An organ generated by desire, and by hunger. It is the embryo's home and lifeline, linking and separating, filtering nutrients and waste. Through the placenta, the mother's body feeds and nourishes the growing fetus, gives the baby blood-borne oxygen until she is thrust out, mouth open, to her first breath and cry, cut free from her flesh anchor. The cord pulses with blood, and then stops, and the placenta is released from the uterus, blood vessels tearing. It is shed, an organ no longer living. A piece of dead meat. Meat for which no animal had to die, but via which, rather, one came to life.

⁘

IN THEIR HOUSE, her husband is the barbecuer, the griller, the preparer of all things dead. Having mastered the intricate boning of salmon and the art of duck confit, he was keen for new culinary challenges, and took her suggestion for the placenta with a degree of professional interest. Skilled at slicing, butchering, filleting, even *he* remarked, once it thawed, that the placenta was fiendishly difficult to cut. It lay on a rimmed cookie sheet, a thick slab of meat the size of four dinner plates stacked together. The top side was ridged with veins and arteries, a road map of the past nine months, all paths leading inevitably to the long, whitish umbilical cord in the center. Then he turned the placenta over, examining it. The bottom side was fleshier, lobed with deep red blobs like ripe plums, wet and sore as a wound.

Even with the sharpest knife, he had to saw at it.

"It's like fish," he said. "A tough outer coating, and inside, soft and then not soft, difficult again."

"But no bones."

"No," he said, studying the bloody terrain. "I suppose not."

She watched as he worked, not quite cutting but pulling the

placenta into bite-sized chunks. With each cut, it oozed blood, type A+, and a liquid she guessed was amniotic fluid. The membrane, the sac in which their daughter had grown, adhered stickily to the bulk of the placenta, or bubbled up with pockets of air and fluid. "Be careful," she admonished as he pulled the membrane away. "This was one of my vital organs."

She couldn't touch it. The chilled clamminess of raw meat made her hands shake. Raw chicken, raw steak, raw liver. This was like liver, and kidneys, and something else besides. Only better. Only worse. Like liver, like kidneys, it was once a living, functioning organ. But it functioned in, belonged to, *her* body, and to the small warm baby sleeping in the next room.

Flesh of our flesh.

·⁘·

THEY WERE HOME from the hospital when her mother arrived at their house, bearing flowers and fruit and scooping up the baby with eager arms. "Look at those yummy cheeks," she cooed. "Oh, I could just eat her up."

"Sure," said her husband, eyes bleary. "I'll find a recipe."

Her mother hugged the baby protectively, but he pressed on. "Really. What if you were given the chance to try human flesh, without anyone having to die?"

Yet unspoken, the word "cannibalism" rang hollow on the kitchen's purple walls, splashed like a grease stain on the tidy dishtowels. She pictured distant jungles on tropical islands, explorers steaming in comic book stewpots. Or remote airplane crashes in snowbound mountains, survivors huddled for warmth under a twisted fuselage, picking the bones of departed fellow travelers.

"Where on earth did you get the idea to eat it?" asked her mother who, despite having given birth to her in the free-swinging '60s, would never have done such a thing.

"It was the cat," she said, holding the baby to her breast, soothing her mewling. Six years old, she had watched a cat birth a litter of tabby kittens, tearing the sacs from each small, wet body, licking them into life. The placentas were attached, small meaty pieces like raw chicken livers, and the mother cat devoured them, growling, a starving animal crouched over fresh kill while the kittens mewed and pushed at its swelling teats.

She thinks of the cat, how it shouted with surprise at the kittens' emergence. The way she herself had squatted, grunted, howled, and pushed.

⁘

ON THE CUTTING board, the placenta is waiting, bleeding into itself.

It's not really cannibalism, she thinks. It's autocannibalism. Self-eating. No different, really, from chewing one's own fingernails.

He is stirring the onions, dividing their sliced layers into strips. "Just consider it a culinary exercise, not a desperate act of survival. You can think like that about cooking anything. Forget about *who* you'd taste. Think about *how* they'd taste."

She has tasted blood, and skin, and sweat, and the syrup of other people's pleasure. That salty tang. Ocean. We're not that far off from animals, really.

"We could just stop here," she says. "Let's not and say we did."

But the meat's finally ready to cook, chopped into small chunks only a centimeter wide and thick. *Diced*, would be the term a chef might use. *Cubed*. Strange, geometric names for something so round and earthy and organic. Clearly inaccurate names for something that solidly resisted every attempt to pare it into uniform pieces.

In their once-vegetarian household, she has agreed to eat, but not prepare, any meat. This is the compromise they've reached, the agreement that came when her pregnant body's need for protein sidled alongside his cravings for a good steak.

"I can't believe *you*, Ms. Veggie Food Freak, are going to eat placenta," said her friend. "You won't even eat fresh fruit if you can't read the ingredients first."

"This is different," she explained. "I know exactly where it's from. I grew it. It's organic."

Before, she had been so devout. No dead animals in *her* kitchen. No processed things she couldn't pronounce, no instant snack foods with lists of ingredients that took longer to read than the food did to eat. No food that made her nervous, like lobster with its snatching claws, sushi with its recent history as glass-eyed fish. No food that gave her itchy lips, or made her fat, or hurt in any way. No food that wasn't organic, free-range, carefully selected and washed and prepared.

She was not a picky eater. She was an obsessively picky eater. She ate for sheer survival, rice, beans, whole grains, and endless lentil stews. Her husband learned macrobiotic, learned tofu, learned miso. Yearned for steak.

But then, with the growing body of evidence that she was becoming nourishment for another person, the balance tipped.

Excellent nutrition is the key to a healthy placenta, and thus a healthy baby, proclaimed her midwife, telling the story of a mother who ate nothing but corn chips and cola. *That* woman's placenta fell apart in the midwife's hands. Ground beef wrapped in tissue.

She began to read. Food books, cookbooks, anything that explained food, its origins, its preparations. And, most importantly, what kinds of nutrients it could offer the swimming fish in her belly. She balanced legumes and grains, added wheat germ and bananas to her protein shakes. She consumed whole milk instead of reduced-fat. She even forgave salmon its rigid, slippery death throes, forgot the horror she'd gathered like muck in the bottoms of boats, and learned to eat it for its omega-3s. All acts of deliberate determination, all calculated to produce a healthy baby.

In her sixth month, with swelling ankles that threatened toxemia, it became clear she couldn't consume enough vegetarian food to keep from becoming dangerously protein-deficient. It was time for blood.

She phoned her husband at work. "I want ribs."

Silence.

"Sweetie?"

Within hours, she found herself heaving her belly through the grocery store's chilled meat section, shivering with anticipation at so many pieces of dead cow, dead pig, dead chicken, all lying there bloody and raw, bones showing through plastic wrap.

The first tentative tastes of ribs were a surprise. Holding the bone end by end, touching her tongue to the sauce, chewing the tender pink meat. She inhaled the aroma of tomatoes and pepper and thought, *Yes, this is good,* and swallowed. Deep inside, the baby kicked with pleasure.

From there, they went to chicken, breaded, sautéed, roasted with hundreds of cloves of garlic inside. And then pork chops with onions and mushrooms, lamb, duck, veal tender with the memory of its womb. And steak, so rare it bled. She ate it all, the world opening through her lips. She lapped the sauces and juices and wanted more.

"Meat, yes, but why placenta?" Her friend was incredulous.

"It's healthy. It has vitamin K, which helps blood clot. It could slow the postpartum flow. It has other nutrients, too, iron and protein and I don't know. Your body makes it. Why not reclaim it? Why break the nutritional circle?"

All of this was simply rationalization. Because the truth of the matter was, she was curious. She wanted a new culinary challenge. She wanted to eat it just to know if she could.

"What would *you* do if you could eat human flesh, without anyone having to die?"

⋰⋱

THE MEAT IS ready to go into the skillet, chunks of deep red flesh that look like the feeling of birth itself.

It sizzles when it hits the hot Teflon. The blood quickly coagulates into cooked protein, while the flesh changes from red and bloody to dull brown and then, as it cooks, mingling with the garlic and onions, to a rich, deep brown, almost black. The smell changes, too, from vegetable to blood, a metallic overtone that hits at the top of her nose. It's definitely meat. Vegetarian meat.

Remember, no animal died for this. Instead, one came to life, and she's sleeping like a lamb in pink pajamas under a cozy bunny-patterned blanket on the futon-couch.

Her husband cuts a piece open to see if it's done. What temperature should it have reached? There are no recipes to adapt, no guidelines to follow. Not even *The Joy of Cooking*, with its recommendations for ptarmigan and whale, offers a simple preparation method or suggests an appropriate spice. So they pretend it's liver, and act accordingly. Inside the cut cube, there's no rawness left, although it's retained a bit of its dark reddish-brown color. If it were liver, it would be done. And indeed, it smells like liver and onions and garlic, and then again, not at all like liver and onions and garlic.

She loves liver and onions and garlic.

Suddenly nervous, she keeps telling herself that's exactly what it is. Repeating it quietly as she lays out placemats and silverware, a centerpiece of white daisies rescued from her withering hospital bouquets. It's liver. It's liver. It's liver. Is there really any difference from one organ to another, one animal to another? When it comes down to it, we're all meat.

He tumbles the food onto two plates, slightly more on hers than on his.

"You are what you eat?" he asks, pulling out her chair. "Or, you eat what you are."

"Were," she says, watching him settle into his seat. "You first. Chef's prerogative."

"No, you. It's your body."

She takes a deep breath, and forks a piece of the garlic first, a slice fried almost crisp. She pauses, then places it on her tongue. She chews. It tastes like fried garlic. Perfectly edible. And then the onions, caramelized to perfection.

"Well?"

"So far, so good."

"Come on, try the meat."

She pokes the smallest piece of placenta onto the tines of her fork. It's springy, as though it's been cooked too long. "How do we know it's cooked right?"

"It's cooked."

"You're sure."

"Come on."

"All right, I'm getting to it."

"I'll get the camera."

Respite. For a moment. He focuses on her mouth, waiting. She feels like a cat backed into a corner.

"Maybe I should check the baby."

"She's fine. Sleeping like a baby."

She opens her lips. The piece of placenta goes into her mouth. She chews, and chews, and slowly, when she's chewed every last bit, carefully swallows.

She is beyond taste, beyond sensation. She feels as though she's again left her body. Gone somewhere else. Become someone else.

"How is it?"

And then, from somewhere in her after-birth euphoria, her post-partum high of hormones and adrenaline and sleep deprivation, she tumbles back to herself, the here and now congealed into a plate of cooked placenta, a shaft of sunlight on her hand, a baby sleeping in the next room, and her husband, watching her with awe. She returns to her body, to decipher the complicated web of flavor and anxiety, to come to terms with the taste of herself.

"It's not bad. Actually, it's good. Needs salt." This surprises her. She'd thought it would have contained saltiness, tasted a little like sweat. It doesn't, so he goes to the kitchen counter and gets some French grey sea salt, and she crumbles a few grains onto the meat. And tastes again. Better. It's like a bland, metallic liver, but springy. Not as dense as calf or chicken liver, nowhere near as rich as *foie gras*. More like kidneys. But different, too. Spongy. In a meaty way.

She chews and swallows again, and nods across the table. "Your turn."

He tastes, chews slowly, swallows. Takes a drink of water. "Not bad. But you need it more than I do."

He dumps his portion onto her plate. She feels an unfamiliar tickle in her throat, an itch, bile rising. She wonders if she could be allergic. Is that possible? There must be some reason for taboos against cannibalism. But autocannibalism?

An hour later, she is still alive. She's eaten the entire plateful, and is hungry again. As she nurses the baby, her husband chops the rest of the raw placenta, fries it with mushrooms and bacon, and whizzes it all in the food processor for a hearty pâté. He tastes it, but that's all. "The rest," he says, "is up to you."

⁕

SHE DOESN'T FINISH the whole Tupperware dish of pâté. After a week of sandwiches, the thick dark-brown spread smeared across whole-grain pumpernickel, she begins to worry about food safety, microbes, invisible toxins.

But she can't just get rid of it—the hospital had clearly stated, handing her a form to sign, that it was a biohazard. A human organ. You can't just throw a placenta in the garbage. If you put it out with the kitchen scraps, you'll be in trouble with the authorities.

"Give it to the dog," her husband nods at their panting chow.

"And have him develop a taste for people?"

But she doesn't want to leave it to grow mold in the refrigerator, either.

"Plant it with the rest," he suggests. They'd frozen the umbilical cord and membrane, parts that couldn't be cooked. She'd already picked out a red rose bush.

She frowns. "You can't put old pâté under a plant."

Eventually, she grinds it up in the garbage disposal, flushing it with gallons of water into the city's sewage system.

Later, the baby nurses, holding her finger in its tiny starfish fist. Flesh of my flesh. She has returned to her body, consuming and consumed.

placenta pâté

a chunk of fresh placenta

½ lb. mushrooms

½ lb. bacon

½ cup mayonnaise

salt and pepper to taste

Fry the bacon until crisp and put aside. Use some of the bacon fat to cook the placenta, in small chunks, until it's not bleeding anymore. Put it aside, sauté the mushrooms in the remaining oil, and whiz all ingredients in a food processor until they're smooth. Chill and serve on toast points or pumpernickel. Keep refrigerated, no longer than a week.

kitchen confessional

{ CHRISTINE SIENKIEWICZ }

Brandied Ricotta: RICOTTA cheese, powdered sugar, brandy, and cinnamon. With an electric mixer, beat together all ingredients. Mound cheese mixture onto a plate. Cover and chill. Serve with fruit. Sounds simple enough. The recipe was in fact selected for its simplicity. But when I arrive home, set down my grocery bags, and gather what I need to prepare this elegant concoction, I realize there is a problem. I don't *have* an electric mixer. I'm not confident that I know precisely what one is. I scour the page for a footnote about alternative machinery. Anxiously I read the introduction and the glossary for any hint of what other apparatus might be used to "beat together" in the absence of a mixer. A whisk? A fork? A blender? . . . But I find nothing. I am at a loss as to how to proceed. I sit for what seems a shameful eternity staring at the beautiful photo of the summer fruits and sweet cheese . . . helpless. As usual when these situations arise, I call my friend

Alice, an excellent cook and a generally kind person, open to answering psychologically revealing questions. She assures me that she has beaten successfully on a number of occasions by wrapping her hand around the handle of a wooden spoon and stirring vigorously. With this jewel of kitchen esoterica, I am able to move forward, and, albeit in twice the time prescribed, finish.

I know what you're thinking, "She didn't know what a mixer was? Come *on*." But it's true. I really didn't know, and I'm an otherwise intelligent, well-rounded person. I play the piano! Ask me about dog breeds, about paint finishes, about medical notation. I have a thing or two to offer, it's just that none of them are edible.

Scenarios such as the ricotta incident are commonplace for the novice cook. In this case, a novice cook who recently has become insecure about being a full-grown self-respecting woman with little or no knowledge of the culinary basics. My skills rival those of can-and-box bachelors who are the butt of many a woman's joke. With the exception of a few first-tier meals from long-bygone college days (stir-fried x, stir-fried y), I simply can't cook.

I'm not sure how it happened, but looking back, I will admit there was an innocent disinterestedness at play from the start. My mother cooked dinner most nights without much fuss, and called the family to the table when it was ready. I certainly enjoyed eating food, but was never terribly concerned with its origin or preparation. There were plenty of other, more interesting curiosities to pursue: bands to front, school plays to star in, stories to pen, canvasses to paint, and, of course, a seemingly infinite number of Atari 2600 cartridges to conquer.

Then, as a young adult, I amassed a group of friends all quite talented in the kitchen. They loved to cook, and enjoyed sharing their creations with someone who was in awe of their passion and ability. They cooked, I ate, and this seemed to work well for everyone.

These same friends were quick to label me, though I didn't take my reputation too seriously. When parties came along, I was the Bring the Drinks Friend. (See also: Bring the Chips Friend.) Once, I set out to host a dinner and invited several people to my apartment. I arranged for my friend Rose to "help" me cook. This meant Rose cooked and I performed discrete support tasks such as chopping an onion or handing off potholders. One guest who chose to socialize in the kitchen and nose around in the meal-preparation dynamics commented, "Christine, it's strange you've made it this far and learned so little about cooking." Rose responded eagerly to augment the point, "Ha! Never mind cooking. She doesn't even know how to *move* in a kitchen." Her vaudevillian reenactment of stiff, confused gestures gave everyone a good chuckle, and she then followed up with a quick feel-good consolation comment about my ability to fix stereo equipment. Sadly, the remark was close to true. Others danced gracefully around a kitchen with an economy of motion that made it look effortless. I needed a map.

There have been times when I've needed to cook. As a student living abroad in Spain I was forced into some amount of cookery as my home was remote by urban standards (no walkable takeout). Fried-egg-and-bologna sandwiches became a staple. But I could never get the egg part quite right. I was frying eggs as a monkey might, mimicking the flipping motions I'd seen other people make. The result was a heap of rubbery overcooked-egg tatters slumped atop one another. My host, a dignified Spanish doña who kept an impeccable house and considered cooking a serious matter, had silently witnessed this spectacle many times while passing through in the background. One day she finally blurted out, *"¡Mira! ¡Christine está cocinando sus famosos huevos muertos!* (Look! Christine is making her famous dead eggs!)"

Every non-cook is full of secret war stories about attempted (failed) and aborted meals. Over the years I collected more than a few. At the same time, my friends were going deeper, advancing into gourmet territory. They seemed to be in it together, on parallel tracks, propagating the notion *en vogue* that cooking prowess was a lofty attribute. An attribute not with overtones of "that was a lovely pot roast, dear"; rather "I'm mesmerized by you, your food makes me weak, I'm melting at your table." Cooking was evolving into high art, and I was being squarely left out.

I would listen to others tell stories of my food follies over flawless meals prepared for me and my boyfriend (of whom I was extremely fond) and they began to make me bristle. Society was making a permanent distinction between those who cooked and those who didn't. My poor showing thus far was going to be a lifelong albatross. The prospect of feeling perpetually deficient in a major life category and being branded as such made me supremely uneasy: Not being able to cook was suddenly a problem. *My* problem. I was envious of people like Rose and Alice. I wanted people to melt at my table too. Then other reasons rose to the surface, strengthening the case. I wanted to be more healthful. I wanted to have more of a relationship with my food. Okay, I wanted to impress my boyfriend. Regardless of the relative importance of the individual reasons, the sum total made me determined to break free from my past, free from the shackles of alimentary ignorance, and learn, not just to cook, but to cook *well*.

At age thirty, with no mentor, this enterprise is not easy. Cooking has a nomenclature, a grammar, more easily assimilated by the young, to the point where what has been learned by those who cook becomes difficult to deconstruct for others. The basic building blocks of cooking that so many take for granted must be explicitly acquired later in life. The novice learning alone is living in a foreign environment with no translator. No question is too elementary, and nothing is instinctive.

"Julienne and blanch ginger." I hated those girls in high school. "Add skate wings to your court bouillon." *What?*

"A tamis for the blini." Okay! And a tambourine for that kid in the back!

Novices need things explained down to the very last pinch of salt. When I was instructed to make spaghetti sauce with "a couple of cans of tomatoes," I was disappointed when I hit the canned tomato aisle that no one had clarified a twenty-four versus a twelve-ounce can, peeled or diced or whole. . . . I required on-call counsel, someone not only willing to entertain these types of facile inquiries, but someone able to answer them plainly and without judgment.

With that resource secured (Alice), the logical place to start was cookbooks. What I didn't fully realize until I got more serious about my undertaking, however, was that cookbooks and recipes assume varying amounts of knowledge (almost always knowledge I do not have). Cookbooks are not unlike auto-repair manuals: If you don't know where the engine is, you're going to have a hard time of it.

Well-intentioned people told me in earnest to "start with easy recipes." Unfortunately, if you don't know how to cook, you can't reliably recognize a simple recipe. Take, for instance, a white sauce. Ignoring the word "roux," white sauce looks reasonably straightforward on paper. Melt butter; stir in flour, milk, pepper; and call it done. I made white sauce from two different recipes, diligently heating the milk, whisking all the while. Both times the sauce was full of lumps, lumps, and more lumps that refused to dissipate and rendered it inedible. I called Alice. She clued me in to the fact that *all* the flour needs to be whisked in *before* the milk. "Solid before liquid," she said—an axiom applicable to many contexts, really. Two recipes and nary a mention of this important sequence.

My extensive experience in this area has led me to believe there should be an independent ratings committee (headed by me) that reviews cookbooks and scores them with a one-to-four spatula rating. One spatula would indicate that instructions are explained in detail appropriate for a beginner. The called-for equipment and ingredients would be either on hand or easily attained. For example: "Plunge beans into a large pot of rapidly boiling water. Cook 5 minutes, or until just tender-crisp. Meanwhile, prepare a large bowl of ice water. Drain beans and plunge into ice water until cool. Drain and pat dry with paper towels." This is known as "refreshing," the recipe tells me, "which stops the cooking instantly and also sets the color." Plain language, directions are broken down into their simplest parts, and indicators of doneness are accompanied by precious time estimates. In my experience homey cookbooks excel in this area—the previous example's helpful hand-holding was provided by the Junior League of Seattle's *Simply Classic* cookbook. At the other end of the spectrum, most celebrity-chef cookbooks merit a four-spatula rating, meaning you should seek a professional's assistance (or Alice) before you proceed. When a recipe instructs me to use a Silpat, to brush with clarified butter, or to cut potatoes with a mandoline, I start to feel faint. I need Silpats spelled out, I need clarification on clarifying, and if I'm going to cut potatoes, I'm pretty sure a banjo would work better than a mandoline.

The crawling phase of learning to cook is filled with many mysteries and frustrations, but none as hairy as food safety. The fact that food preparation involves principles of chemistry and biology is extraordinarily intimidating. These are forces beyond our control and often our ken, forces that have the power to maim and kill. Food ingredients known to carry these risks strike the fear of God in me. (Perhaps this is why I was "vegetarian"—wherever meat, substitute cheese—for a few years.) If, for instance, a recipe calls for marinating in a nonreactive pan it is quickly cast aside, not only because I'm not sure what kind of pan that would be, but moreover because if the chemical risks are overtly stated, it's too risky for me.

A few years ago, I was tapped to contribute to the office potluck.

My assignment was "side dish." I decided on something safe, a dish I had successfully made at least once before: black bean salad with corn, red pepper, onion, cilantro, cumin, and lemon juice. I remembered it as being relatively easy and tasting like it was harder to make than it was, a key criterion for potluck entries. I tossed it together on the eve of the event and carried it in with confidence the next day. Partway through the luncheon, a coworker asked who made it, and when my boss pointed to me she came to tell me in person how delicious it was. Then she asked, with wide eyes and an impish yet collegial smile, "Christine, this is great. When did you find time to soak beans?"

A bystander joined in: "I was thinking the same thing. I'm so beat when I get home I can hardly make a sandwich."

Soak beans? Was I supposed to soak beans?

"No kidding," continued the first. "Now that I'm working full-time, I only get to shop once a week . . ." The two pattered on while my mind began to race. I had used black beans straight from the can and not thought twice of it. Was there some toxic compound from the metal that had to be cooked out? I immediately catastrophized the situation. I envisioned the roomful of oblivious partygoers, mouths brimming with bean salad, smiling and laughing as they turned green and fell to the floor one by one.

I excused myself, swiftly exited the building, and called Alice. She informed me that I had in fact done no harm; rather I had been the victim of some Berkeley Natural Foodies' expectations. And although in the BNF paradigm, using non-organic produce or canned beans may have been disconcerting and politically incorrect, it proved no threat to anyone's health.

For the novice cook, preparing food for others is always a trying experience. Early on I learned to think of cooking a meal for a guest as a unit by which to measure trauma: two to four hours with significant increase in heart rate, onset of ulcer, and a post-meal lingering melancholy. The novice is slow, messy, nervously juggling a meal's components while anticipating the worst possible outcomes. I had such unpleasant experiences trying to cook for people that the prospect of doing it on a regular basis had always seemed repugnant. To note:

- ❖ OCCASION: Father's Day. Menu: pesto halibut and new potatoes. Total preparation time: two hours. Result: undercooked, parasitic playground (despite the fact that I sought out instructions, used a ruler to measure the thickest part of the fish, and set its cooking time accordingly).
- ❖ OCCASION: Parents over to new apartment. Menu: chile-cheese casserole. Total preparation time: two hours. Result: intestinal masonry.
- ❖ OCCASION: First Thanksgiving (turkeyless) for self and ex. Menu: stuffed zucchini, tomato bisque, and Waldorf salad. Total preparation time: four hours. Result: Actually, the food was okay, but the ex was totally disassociative, inhaled the meal in less than twenty minutes, and then claimed he was tired and went to bed. Traumatic, *bien sur*.

More recently, I made an onion *tarte Lyonnaise*. It called for a *pâte brisée*, "the shortest of the short crusts." I had never made a crust before, but from what little I'd observed of my mother's pie-making, this one seemed suspiciously crumbly. I had to work to get it into a cohesive whole covering the bottom of the pie dish. Onion, cheese, egg, cream, butter, nutmeg, salt, and pepper made the filling, but when the tart was done, the half-inch of dry, grainy crust with its utilitarian flavor was too dominant and overpowered the dish. I had made my short crust too tall! That seemed a forgivable offense. Next time I would simply make the crust thinner, or use a different pastry.

The tart, although imperfect, was a surprisingly painless experience and marked a shift in my experience of cooking. It didn't seem so difficult. Where before I felt as if I were corralling ingredients together by force, combining and cooking them against their will, I now am beginning to feel some sense of understanding. Food is not the enemy. I can make informed choices based on comprehensible mistakes, and control different outcomes. Aside from being more inspired, I am cooking with a frequency that actually allows what I learn to build on itself. Things are starting to gel.

Now when I go to friends' houses for dinner, I actually *pay attention*. Most of them are happy to narrate a meal's preparation and answer questions. Occasionally something goes wrong, and fixes involve a bit of improvisation and guesswork. It's reassuring to know that even good cooks can ruin a dish! A communal fallibility of sorts.

Even in the short time that I've been working on my cooking, progress is evident. Questions are less often necessary, and a few recent ones weren't so easy for even the experts to answer. The four-spatula recipes, although too difficult to undertake, aren't looking as much like foreign-language texts. I'm starting slowly, but ever striving toward the canapés from the *French Laundry*. Along with my own rehabilitation, I am retraining my friends and family to think of me as a normal person, with cooking potential. Armed with a sizable newfound confidence (and Alice), cooking seems not only doable, but alluring. Someday perhaps I will be the recipient of those phone calls that begin, "Hi, it's me again. I have a cooking question . . ." I vow to answer plainly and without judgment.

paddington's marmalade, jo's apples

{ KAREN ENG }

ALMOST MORE THAN I love food, I love to read. So it follows that I love reading about food. There's something exceedingly pleasant about the sensation of words firing my food-related synapses, and, to me, the discussion of food, particularly among friends and family, provides a peculiar satisfaction that neither food nor words alone can provide. As M.F.K. Fisher wrote: "So it happens that when I write of hunger, I am really writing about love and the hunger for it . . . and warmth and the love of it and the hunger for it . . . and then the warmth and richness and fine reality of hunger satisfied . . . and it is all one." This epigraph opens each issue of *PekoPeko*, a zine about food that I publish—the culmination of my lifelong absorption with the written word's relationship to food.

❖

MY ATTACHMENT TO the words-and-food connection began when I was a child and a serious and voracious reader. One of the glories of the Southern Californian summer was the endless stretch of hours I used to do nothing but read, anything I wanted. (My happy memories are only somewhat marred by those of parents— fearful that "too many fiction books" would rot my brain, which would lead me to a vapid life—insisting on "scheduling" once-a-day independent academic study, piano practice, and typing lessons.) At least once a week, I'd visit my local public library, a one-story, air-conditioned, fluorescent-lit cinderblock building that sat right behind the Thrifty drugstore, where they served ice cream cones for a dime. Elaine, the children's librarian, took her job seriously and held her young charges in high regard. Each week, after conferring with her about which books I'd already read and what I was looking for, I'd take out a tall stack—at least ten at a time— devour them all, and come back for more.

Throughout my adulthood I've found myself turning back to those books I read as a kid, making a point to collect my favorites when I come across them in secondhand bookstores, especially in particularly handsome editions or, better yet, in the edition in which I first read them. (My newly acquired paperbacks of *Harriet the Spy* and *A Bear Called Paddington* are soft and tattered, but they're just like the ones I had, and just looking at the covers makes me happy.) Not many adults feel the need to surround themselves with the storybooks of their youth, so why do I? Recently, looking over these small volumes, I realized that most of them have one thing in common—they use food as a central storytelling element.

It's not that I automatically love *any* narrative involving food. The stories that live in my taste buds are those that drew me into a world I could not have otherwise known, books written so vividly, I could swear I've drunk hot maple sugar fresh from the tree, or known what it feels like to catch a drop of peach juice on my tongue—from the inside of the peach! Though I haven't done those things, I don't need to, because I've experienced them again and again through reading.

In the limited world of the child, books are a way to be transported, and these books allowed me to travel beyond my own gastronomical reality. Mine wasn't boring: I grew up in an immigrant Chinese family, in a little California dairy town called Cypress. This meant trips to Los Angeles Chinatown for shopping expeditions that included watching chickens get their throats slit and thrown into metal garbage cans to thrash with a terrible banging while bleeding to death, dim sum and luxurious banquets around tables with my vast extended family, and chewy, glutinous dumplings that disappeared from the table when my grandparents grew too old to make them.

But it also meant pork chops, Thanksgiving stuffing, and prime rib that couldn't be beat, thanks to my grandfather's early career as a Western-style cook when he first came to this country. It meant bushels of huge, sun-warmed strawberries from the fields next to our 1970s housing tract. It meant corn dogs from the food court at the mall, latkes and gefilte fish at my best friend's house two doors down, Otter Pops by the pool. And the years our family spent in Taiwan offered even more memorable experiences: plain rice porridge for breakfast, accompanied by little dishes of savory condiments; blood sausage; "stinky" tofu; white corn; hot soy milk I'd bring home in a bucket from a stand to eat with fry bread; star fruit, longan; and fruits that don't even have names in English. All this and more made up my childhood gastronomical vocabulary, and I use them as signposts, anchoring me to time, place, and relationships.

Slowly, I became aware that the food people eat and the way they choose to procure, prepare, and share it reveals much about who they are, where they come from, and what they value. My grandmother, for instance, who grew up in Burma and Hong Kong, ate Jacob's Cream Crackers from a blue tin and sometimes put milk in her tea (something my grandmother from China would never do)—which told some part of my consciousness that she came from a British colony and lived through an era affected by wartime frugality. Food became how I decoded the world around me, and that must have extended to the worlds only my imagination had access to. In any narrative, but even more so in children's literature, food is the magic key that allows access to, and a way to interpret, other worlds. It's a point of empathy as well as of strangeness, sometimes simultaneously: We can all relate to hunger.

And just as I hunt down dim sum on Saturday mornings to fill up on the familiar, I fumble for certain children's books at my bedside whenever I need to remember the flavors that captured my young fancy.

⸫

PROBABLY THE FIRST historical novels many of us ever read, the Little House books provided a wealth of information on how American settlers survived on the frontier in the 1870s and '80s. More important, they brought home the concept—entirely foreign to my comfortable, 1970s suburban life—that there was such a thing as a struggle for one's daily bread, that "working" means something far more extensive than going to the office every day to make money for groceries.

In the Little House books, life revolves around getting food on the table. From morning to night, according to Wilder's account, the family of five set about feeding, milking, farming, churning, slaughtering, cooking—a roster of activities that didn't leave time for much else. When *my* mom wanted fresh fish, we'd pry ourselves away from the TV long enough to get in the car and drive the quarter mile to Thrif-T-Mart or Albertson's, or, on special occasions, visit the fishing boats that pulled into Newport Beach on the weekend. Pa Ingalls, however, set fish traps under one of Plum Creek's waterfalls. If we wanted fresh meat, we'd buy it from the supermarket or butcher. Pa hunted game animals whose numbers had to be minded so that they wouldn't fall too low. Butter? Unwrap ice-cold blocks from the fridge. When the Ingallses needed butter, they took a day to churn it. If we wanted salt or sugar, we could buy it anywhere for pennies. The Ingallses traveled far to trade furs they'd trapped for these precious commodities, which were used as sparingly as saffron and vanilla beans are now.

All this was new and exotic to me. While I knew I was growing up in a culture where the Ingallses' odyssey constituted a historical reality, my own ancestors didn't actually experience American pioneer life as Wilder tells it, and neither did my best friend's, or anyone else's, as far as I knew. My family had farmed, yes, but in another country, in a culture far removed. I wasn't consciously aware of the gap, but if I had thought about it, I would have realized that my parents and grandparents still tilled soil and planted vegetables and fruits in our backyard, from which we often ate, and that when we bought chickens from the Chinese butcher they were killed just for us. Looking back, my life wasn't quite as far removed from the Ingallses' labor-to-table lifestyle as I had imagined.

Paradoxically, I absorbed the lessons from the Little House series more easily than I handled my own family's memories of fleeing war and starvation in Asia. Maybe it was because the culture of Little House seemed less remote; maybe the lack of distance from my own family's history was too intense for a kid to process. Easier to wonder what happens to the flavor of the cow's milk when she's starving because of a plague of grasshoppers, and to think about how domestic animals must be cared for daily regardless of blizzards or, even when regarded as affectionately as pets, must be slaughtered for the meat that would allow the family to survive through winter. Though probably harrowing at times, such a life, viewed from a distance, is oddly romantic. With faith and work, people can survive the wilderness. And even simple things should not be taken for granted.

Particularly magical are Wilder's descriptions of sweets, one of very few luxuries in her childhood, with which she was clearly enthralled. In *Little House in the Big Woods*, Laura and her sister make Christmas candy by pouring a cooked molasses mixture in pans of snow and letting it harden. Later, at a winter maple-sugar gathering at her grandfather's Wisconsin home, they boil down a huge iron kettle of sap tapped from the trees overnight before pouring it out to harden into dark cakes of crumbly sugar (used for "common every day," in contrast to white, "store-bought," which was only set out for special occasions). At the party the children gather clean snow from outdoors to cool the hot syrup into soft candy— a process that seemed exquisitely sensual to me—while the grownups inside dance to the fiddle.

Growing up in Southern California, I had plenty of access to sugar of all kinds, but not to real snow. I longed to make snow angels like Laura and Mary. But my sister and I did, more than once, approximate the maple-sugar candy to the best of our ability with our toy Sno-Cone kit. First we'd shave away at a block of ice with a shaver built into a molded-plastic bird with earmuffs. We'd then dump the shaved ice into a cup and squirt Log Cabin syrup (which we thought was actual maple syrup) into it—and the results were always disappointing. Sweet, slushy, and watery, the syrup mixed into the ice and never formed into a mass that we could pull out and eat.

But my favorite passage from the Little House books is from *On the Banks of Plum Creek*, when Nellie Oleson's mother serves a group of girls a "white sugar cake" and lemonade at Nellie's birthday party. It keenly describes a girl's first taste of refined flavors and her response: "'Is your lemonade sweet enough?' Mrs. Oleson asked. So Laura knew that it was lemonade in the glasses. She had never tasted anything like it. At first it was sweet, but after she ate a bit of the sugar-white off her piece of cake, the lemonade was sour."

·❖·

AT AROUND THE same time in history, but leading a vastly different based-on-reality life of sacrifice and determination, the Alcott sisters were growing up in the civilized environs of Concord, Massachusetts. When I first read *Little Women*, I had no context for it. I didn't even know then that it was the Civil War that kept Mr. March away from home (I don't think the book ever names it). Now I read *Little Women* yearly, usually when winter begins and I want to cozy up in bed with a book, and with each reading I discover something new—nuances of emotion, feminist undertones, striking phrases I was once too young to register.

Like Little House, the Little Women books are about survival in the face of hardship, though the latter family had once known wealth and was simply struggling through a difficult time. In *Little Women*, food represents sharing as well as deprivation—and illustrates the social humiliation poverty brings. The girls miss the fancy things they enjoyed years before and must content themselves with simpler fare. Even so, charity comes first: When Marmee asks the girls to give up their Christmas breakfast to a destitute family, they muster their compassion and spend the morning doing the good deed, later eating plain bread and milk when they get home. Later that day, their kindness is rewarded by a feast of sweets sent by the rich old man next door.

In another memorable chapter, Amy wheedles "rag money" from Meg to buy pickled limes, a treat that gains her social currency at school. For a short time Amy enjoys freedom from the embarrassment of poverty, but when she gets caught with the contraband item, she suffers public humiliation resulting from her lack of self-esteem.

I was both repulsed and fascinated by the idea of the limes (I've still never seen or heard of anything like them), and I could empathize with Amy's need to fit in. (Even in the '70s you had to have the "right" sweets: Bubble Yum, Freshen Up, dehydrated apple chips.) But of course I, like most readers, connected most with Jo. What tomboy who wants to grow up to be a writer could ever forget Jo's retreats into the attic with a book, a pile of apples at hand? Apples became romantic, a symbol of the writer's solitary, melancholy life, something one wants to have a bowl of in that room of one's own. Because one can munch through them thoughtfully, sustaining oneself without having to get up and prepare a meal, they also symbolize focus. Recently, when I rented my own office for the first time, I christened it with a bowl of apples on the table. I didn't eat most of them . . . I have to be in the mood for apples, and they have to be just so. But I simply didn't feel right until they were there.

Little Women's sense of deprivation thankfully disappears in Alcott's sequel, *Little Men,* in which Jo has found her calling as the matron of a boys' school. The smells of an idyllic childhood haven are plentiful here: "shiny" gingerbread, pies, fresh bread—wholesome, plain, nourishing food. And, of course, apples. Here Jo is in her element: a lone woman nurturing a sea of boys, echoed by the presence of young tomboy student Nan. Meg's daughter Daisy is also here, though she's a more traditional girl. Nan can get as rough as the boys, but Daisy becomes bored and wants to play in the kitchen with the cook, giving her Aunt Jo an idea. Through Uncle Laurie, Jo procures a fully functional iron stove, along with pots, pans, a coal bin, dishes, and "two doll's pans of new milk, with cream actually rising on it, and a wee skimmer all ready to skim it with"—putting our Easy-Bake Ovens to shame. The vivid description of Daisy's first miniature pie-baking, squash-mashing, and steak-broiling attempts are so delicious, I was almost tempted as a kid to try it, but the urge ended there. It wasn't a yen for gender equality that stopped me: I preferred to sit in my room reading to cooking, and the kitchen was my mother's domain, anyway. What if she made me do the dishes?

A COUPLE OF days ago a friend who has known me for over a decade affectionately accused me of being an Anglophile. Reflecting on why I might cherish such familial feelings for the British Isles when neither I nor my parents were born there, it occurs to me again that my mother and her family were once subjects of the Empire, and, like it or not, the inflections of its language and culture and food—like the tea with milk and cream crackers—made their way into my young consciousness. While my first language was Chinese, my first exposure to English was through my mother, who was taught the Queen's. As much as my fondness for growing my own food must have come from the farming background of my father's parents, and the comfort I take in my local Jewish deli must have come from my childhood neighbors, likewise, the promise of a cup of tea and a slice of buttered toast can conjure a warmth I wish I had access to more often.

So it's not surprising that, while *A Bear Called Paddington* is merely a story about a lost bear from an exotic locale finding a home where the normal is extraordinary, it's one I turn to when I want that snug sensation. Mr. and Mrs. Brown, a middle-class London couple, are at Paddington Station picking up their daughter Judy, who is coming home from school for the summer. Mr. Brown notices among the parcels a small brown bear wearing a hat and a label that says "Please look after this bear. Thank you." Turns out he has emigrated—stowed away in a lifeboat and surviving on marmalade—from "Darkest Peru," where his Aunt Lucy has gone to live in a home for retired bears. (My husband, who spent part of his childhood in Lima, assures me there are no bears in Peru.)

As he looks very small and has no place to go, the Browns invite him to stay with them for a while.

Paddington's main relationship to food is one of deep affection and mishap—much like his relationship to the Browns. When he's not getting grapefruit juice in his eye or dropping marmalade sandwiches from the theater balcony onto people's heads below, he is trailing a large piece of bacon salvaged from breakfast in his suitcase, causing dogs to follow him in the London Underground, perplexing Mrs. Brown. When performing a magic trick at his birthday party (the cake contains a cream and marmalade filling), he accidentally conjures a pot of marmalade beneath a crotchety guest's seat. Almost the only time Paddington exhibits dominion over food is when he has begun to assimilate comfortably, shopping for the family in Portobello Road, squeezing fruits for the "right degree of firmness." (This sentence was a revelation to me as a child. It had never occurred to me to squeeze fruit for ripeness.)

Paddington was also my introduction to marmalade, the bear's favorite food, which figures prominently in his life with the Browns. I decided to try it on this basis, in spite of my intense dislike of orange peel in every other context. I don't remember the first time I had it—maybe in college. For years I convinced myself I liked it, even getting into lemon marmalade for a while before I was forced to admit to myself that I was letting jars of it go bad in the fridge, and that in fact I liked the *idea* of preserves—fantasizing about hoarding pots of jam in my pantry when I would finally have my own apartment—much more than I liked the actual stuff.

But more importantly, *Paddington* was my introduction to the extra-extra-dry humor of that part of the world. In the introductory chapter, for example, Mr. Brown, taking into consideration Paddington's love of marmalade, buys him the biggest and stickiest bun he can find, which Paddington decides he must tackle on top of the table. Before long, he's covered in cream and jam and has a tumble-down accident with a cup of hot tea. When Mrs. Brown finds him, she remarks, "You wouldn't think that anyone could get in such a state with just one bun." It's my favorite line in the book, opening the way for a somewhat obnoxious love of Monty Python and (less obnoxiously) Richard E. Grant, whose chicken-killing, eel-poaching antics in *Withnail and I* take the food-mishap comedy into a very adult realm.

In a similar vein, J.R.R. Tolkien's *The Hobbit* and *The Lord of the Rings* presented a deep and tempting sense of comfort in the world of hobbits. From the first "In a hole in the ground there lived a hobbit . . . " I could feel myself drawn through that round green door into a fantasy world that seemed so real, I actually half-believed in it.

As with Paddington, the full-pantry, warm-fire world of Bilbo Baggins represents middle-class normalcy, but in this case is the jumping-off point for adventure rather than the point of arrival. When the dwarves begin appearing in small bunches on Bilbo's doorstep, he's obliged, according to the rules of hospitality, to invite them in and feed them. The writing is delectable and wry: "He found himself scuttling off . . . to the cellar to fill a pint beer-mug, and then to a pantry to fetch two beautiful round seed-cakes which he had baked that afternoon for his after-supper morsel. . . . Bilbo plumped down the beer and the cake in front of them, when loud came a ring at the bell again, and then another ring."

Hobbits are even more preoccupied—and much more adept—with food than Paddington, and as *The Hobbit* and its sequel are primarily from these creatures' point of view, descriptions of their meals practically dictate the rhythm of their journey. From the safety of home—represented by the seed-cake, raspberry jam, pork-pie, salad, beer, and coffee the dwarves demand from Bilbo's pantry—to roasting bits of rabbit and sheep for an emergency cliff-top meal after being rescued from goblins by eagles, to mushrooms, cram, lembas, mead, and coney stew on the interminable road to Mount Doom, *The Hobbit* and *The Lord of the Rings* are essentially very long, dangerous walks punctuated by meals, or worry over where the next meal will come from. The message: There may be more important things in life than a well-stocked larder and a comfortable table, but few things are more desirable. Hobbits are my kind of people.

⋰⋱

AS I WRITE this I'm realizing that while the American books I most enjoyed described situations based in reality, the books by British authors describe fantasy worlds grounded in the familiar, symbolized by food. The realm of comfort is a gateway to adventure —Mary Poppins's gingerbread comes to mind, as does James's peach. In fact, I could mention at least a dozen more children's titles my memory still fondly associates with food—*Heidi, Ozma of Oz, All-of-a-Kind Family, A Wrinkle in Time*, to name a few—and I'm sure, as you read this, that you're generating long lists of your own. I'm deeply indebted to all these stories: My early immersion in them probably makes up a good part of the philosophical foundation on which I built *PekoPeko*, which is more about our complex relationship to food and the worlds it opens up than about the food itself. To my delight and amazement, people have responded very warmly to *PekoPeko*. According to my own professed worldview, I guess I shouldn't be surprised, but readers are often isolated characters, and it's nice to look up from the pages and find I'm not alone with my marmalade fantasies.

mandelbrot memories,
or the bargain hunter

{ DEBRA MEADOW }

"Biscotti, schmiscotti," my grandmother Florence would have declared, with a dismissive wave of her hand and her nose wrinkled in disapproval. "Have some mandelbrot. Eat, eat!"

And eat I did. Brisket, kugel, matzo ball soup, kreplach, and blintzes were the fare at her table, but the treat that transports me back to her kitchen—and her to mine—is mandelbrot. Literally "almond bread," mandelbrot is a dry, twice-baked cookie for dipping, studded with almonds, candied fruit, or—in a New World twist—chocolate chips.

"Now," you may say, "that sounds an awful lot like those cookies for dunking sold from imported jars in designer coffee shops." Well, they may exude the essence of someone's adored Italian nana, but mandelbrot, biscotti's country cousin, contains my bubbe's soul.

Food and feeding are to any immigrant Jewish grandmother as sunlight is to a flower: *it doesn't hurt* (must be said with correct, rising inflection). One fall weekend twenty years ago, my spirits and my book bag dampened by the incessant Northwest rain, I flew south to Phoenix for a long weekend break from college. Grandma—ample and aproned—greeted me at her apartment door, a portal between worlds: Outside were the palms, pools, and hard Southwest sun, but once across the threshold it was all mothball-scented, musty blue, "early New Jersey" décor.

Grandma was pink with purpose because she could simultaneously ply me with food and with questions about the *goyishe* man I had announced I would marry. She sought information—clues she could piece together to answer the question: Was this the end of the world as she knew it? She would gather evidence over the weekend to come, and arrange it just so on the white damask dining room tablecloth to form a picture of just how irreparably I might be damaging my life and severing the unbroken chain of our family's Jewish lineage.

"Olson," she said—again with the wrinkled nose—as she ladled golden chicken soup with kreplach, the Jewish version of won tons, into shallow Limoges bowls I would someday inherit. "What kind of a name is that?"

"His father's family is from Sweden." I cringed, but my trepidation was buffered by melt-in-your-mouth beef brisket, braised the day before with potatoes and onions, chilled overnight, then sliced and reheated in Reynolds Wrap.

"Ach. The Swedes. They drink." Again, she swatted at some invisible irritant. "Does he like your cooking?" she asked, arriving quickly at the crux of the matter.

"Yes, Grandma. I even make oatmeal from scratch." I knew it would impress her in this era of the instant.

If she couldn't find reason, or ammunition, to dissuade me from this reprehensible act she would do the thing she did best: feed me body and soul, so that at least I could carry recipes, if not pure bloodlines, into the future. Her grandchildren must be raised on gefilte fish and chopped liver, not lutefisk and Jell-O salads with mayonnaise.

She carved out a triangle of warm apple pie.

"Ahhh. A bargain he's getting."

⁕

LATER THAT WEEKEND we sat at her table dipping golden slices of mandelbrot, flecked with candied fruit in traffic-light hues, into cups of hot tea. Our ancestors would have taken the tea in a glass sieved through a cube of sugar clenched in their teeth. As I packed to return to school after three days of nudging and nurturing, she plied me with a *pekl*—a small package—of the cookies. "Something for the trip," she explained, as if I were boarding a stagecoach instead of a two-hour flight, to Oregon.

This, as it happens, is mandelbrot's raison d'être. Because the sweet breads are baked first as a log, then cooled, sliced, and briefly toasted in the oven, they keep beautifully for days and even weeks. They made handy, portable snacks for itinerant Old World rabbis and merchants and are perfect for sending in care packages to granddaughters at college, where they arrive delicious and welcomed, if a little battered from shipping.

Because they are baked with oil—rather than with butter, like biscotti are—mandelbrot are also *pareve*—neither meat nor dairy, and can be served with either one in a kosher household where the two are never mixed at a single meal. Though, in a quick Internet search of modern mandelbrot recipes, I found the tally running neck and neck between those made with oil and infidel versions with butter or—horrors!—margarine. Also, mandelbrot usually spend less time in the oven than their Italian counterparts during the second baking, and are moister as a result.

My uncle once declared cinnamon raisin bagels a "culture

shonda"—a shame on the culture. I'm afraid my grandmother would feel the same about chocolate orange mandelbrot. To her, they would be kreplach in ravioli's clothing. But time and innovation march on and I have fussed with her tradition, to delicious result.

No one, not even Grandma, could talk me out of getting married the following year, but they were somewhat mollified that the rabbi who joined us in holy matrimony would only do the deed if we agreed to raise our children as Jews. We are.

Years after our wedding, I found out that in the car on the way to the temple odds were being laid by my uncle as to how long this dubious union would last. Three years? Five? The only thing more counter to tradition was, perhaps, a cinnamon raisin bagel. I think back on this, after almost twenty-two years of marriage, with only a smidgen of moral superiority.

Grandma died sixteen years ago at eighty-eight. She lived just long enough to meet the person she most longed for in her later years, her first great grandchild, my daughter Leah. She would *kvell*, or swoon with pride, to see her at sixteen: beautiful beyond compare, teaching Sunday school in our little congregation, learning about physics and Latin and reading Elie Wiesel. She'd be less happy to learn that my children turn up their noses at gefilte fish, even the homemade kind I prepare each year at Passover in a devoted act of ancestor worship. I've never placed chopped liver within smelling distance of Leah and Sam. They would rather clean the cat box, for heaven's sake, but they do adore matzo ball soup, latkes, and the occasional cheese blintz. They've never heard of lutefisk. They love Jell-O, but hold the mayo, please.

Through cooking, Grandma planted a seed of the mother culture in a new land and a new generation. I remember and savor dozens of her dishes, but it is mandelbrot—the toasty, sweet smell as it comes from the oven and the sandy way it crumbles on my tongue—that summons Grandma to the kitchen chair beside me. We share tea and cookies while my husband washes up the baking pans.

By the third dunk into my cup I can almost hear it: "He washes the dishes, cleans the floors, *and* does the laundry?"

"Ach, you got a bargain."

traditional mandelbrot

3 eggs

¼ cup sugar

1 cup vegetable oil

Zest of 1 lemon, grated or minced

Zest of 1 orange, grated or minced

1 tsp. vanilla extract

¼ tsp. salt

1 T. baking powder

4 cups all-purpose flour

1 cup whole blanched almonds or chopped mixed candied fruit

Beat the eggs and sugar until pale yellow in color. Add the oil, lemon and orange zest, vanilla extract, and salt and beat until well mixed. Mix in the flour and baking powder and gently fold in the almonds or candied fruit.

Turn dough out onto a lightly floured board and gather into a ball. Divide the dough in two equal portions and roll each one into a log, approximately 13 inches long and 2½ inches in diameter. If the dough is sticky, rub a little oil on your hands.

Place the logs onto a well-oiled baking sheet or one lined with parchment paper, leaving space between to allow for spreading. Bake in a preheated 350° oven for about thirty minutes, or until lightly browned. Remove to a rack to cool.

When the logs are completely cool, slice them on the

diagonal into half-inch thick cookies using a serrated bread knife and a gentle sawing motion.

Place slices, cut side up, on the baking sheet and bake in a preheated 400° oven for fifteen minutes, turning the cookies over after seven or eight minutes, or until golden brown on both sides. Watch them carefully, as they burn quickly.

Cool on a rack and store in a tightly sealed container. Makes about thirteen dozen.

chocolate orange mandelbrot

3 eggs

1 cup sugar

1 cup vegetable oil

½ tsp. orange oil, or the grated zest of one large orange

(orange oil will yield a more intense orange flavor)

1 tsp. vanilla extract

¼ tsp. salt

3¼ cups all-purpose flour

¾ cup cocoa powder

1 T. baking powder

1 cup chocolate chips

Beat together eggs and sugar until light yellow in color. Add the oil, orange oil or zest, vanilla, and salt and beat until well mixed. In another bowl blend together the flour, cocoa and baking powder. Add the dry ingredients to the wet mixture and beat until well mixed. Fold in the chocolate chips.

Turn the dough onto a lightly floured board and gather it into a ball. Divide the dough in two equal parts and form each into a log, approximately 13 inches long and 2½ inches in diameter.

Place the logs onto a well-oiled baking sheet or one lined with parchment paper, leaving space between to allow for spreading. Bake in a preheated 350° oven for about thirty minutes. Remove to a rack to cool.

When the logs are completely cool, slice them on the diagonal into half-inch thick cookies using a serrated bread knife and a gentle sawing motion.

Place slices, cut side up on the baking sheet and bake in a preheated 400° oven for fifteen minutes, turning once after seven or eight minutes. Watch them carefully, as they burn quickly.

Cool· on a rack and store in a tightly sealed container. Makes about three dozen.

on the importance of having a restaurant

{ KATE SEKULES }

THIS WILL SURPRISE nobody, but when I left London in 1989 it wasn't the hotbed of food porn it is today. The most daring sandwich in regular circulation was bacon and avocado. A famous French chef had just opened a restaurant without a kitchen and you could get pickled eggs or pork scratchings in any pub, but rarely wine. Ambitious restaurants did exist. One of the most popular —though I think it was on its last legs at that moment—served only appetizers and desserts, the inevitable successor to the tragic era of sliced kiwi fruit and small bundles of *haricots verts* tied with chive string on large black hexagonal plates. London was rather sad then, and the restaurant situation had a lot to do with it—ten years of Margaret Thatcher was the root. But the so-called Iron Lady and her so-called Nanny State, with its dire effects on the capital city, were what I was fleeing, not the inadequacy of the restaurants. Aside from the dearth of pavement tables, and the weather that prohibited them, I liked the London restaurant situation very much, because I had my own place.

It was an intimate, elegantly minimal yet merry joint near where I grew up. I didn't own it. It belonged—still does—to my good friend Jan Woroniecki, a photographer who, due to some arcane lease problem, had to save the family house by opening a restaurant in the bottom of it in 1986. Being one of the heirs to the Polish throne (should such a thing still exist), and son of the late *patron* of Chez Krysthof (the inheritance of which had led to the lease problem), he named it Wódka and invented the first ever *modern Polish* menu. The food, cooked by an intermittently deranged genius whose English was scanty and who occasionally threatened Jan with a meat cleaver, was divine—comfort food ten years ahead of the trend; gutsy posh peasant food in a city of hushed dining rooms and snob chefs who didn't let you salt their dishes. Always on that menu were smoked eel with capers and new potatoes, *golonka* (roast pork shank), *kulebiak* (salmon *en croûte*), and *zrazy* (beef olives). There were fishcakes as good as Le Caprice's, with dill sauce; chicken Kiev, long before trendy foodie irony; and the best *barszcz* (borscht!) in the West. The pierogies were stuffed not with potato but with cheese and almond, or wild mushrooms and sauerkraut, and the buckwheat blini came with smoked salmon or herring or aubergine mousse or, whenever possible, caviar.

It wasn't just the menu I loved, because, of course, good food is only the first prerequisite of a restaurant's success. Other essential factors must work just as well, interwoven into a single alchemical reaction to be repeated night after night. Wódka got all that right. Staff, ambiance, efficiency, location, music, personality, customers, kindness, pricing, and, in this case, vodka, were juggled invisibly, and the restaurant gelled from the first. Early regulars included Jerry Hall and David Bowie, but it was emphatically not a celeb-spotting place (which is probably why they liked it); no, it was a neighborhood place, even if some of the neighbors drove half an hour to reach it. For me, it was even more. It was a wish granted: my home restaurant.

I always wanted one. I was a lucky kid, restaurant-wise. My father, born in '20s Vienna (and Jewish, which I didn't know until five years after he died, but that's another story), was an early prototype of today's foodie. Every January he would start researching that summer's route to the South of France—which Michelin-starred restaurant in the Hautes-Pyrénées was worth a two-day detour (and my map-reader and translator mother's sanity); which obscure Loire Valley vineyards to visit; which hotels in which bourgeois *villes* to stop in. I hated the damn dank wine cellars, loved the crumbly hotels, and adored the restaurants. All the restaurants in the world were in France then (apart from Lyon's Corner House, which was near Charing Cross Station), so in order to choose, my father invented the sport of menu-bashing. We'd arrive at hotel, leave mother in room, walk streets, read menus posted outside restaurants, pick winner, collect mother, have dinner. My menu French was extremely advanced for my age. I also learned to read dining rooms: Cheeses, runny? Linens, starched? Ambiance, confident? Good. Eventually, we'd reach our annual destination, a village on the Côte d'Azur—which sounds posh, but was really quite modest—and that evening be greeted like the long-lost regulars we were at La Reserve in nearby Sainte-Maxime. I would have *tomates provençales, tarte tropézienne,* and diluted *rouge ordinaire.* Now, needless to say, La Reserve remains in memory the Platonic ideal of the home restaurant. I believe we all have one of these. It could be the local IHOP, or the Whistle Stop Cafe, or your nonna's trattoria in Palermo, it doesn't matter as long as it's yours.

Though restaurants exist ostensibly to satisfy hunger, the deepest hunger they're really satisfying is the basic one for community. They provide, temporarily, the extended family and friends that we wish surrounded us. A restaurant is a self-selecting society. Potential customers read between the lines of its menu (*marinara sauce*—old-fashioned, cozy, wear jeans; *roasted tomato-tomatillo salsa*—hip night out, little black dress; *San Marcellano jam with olio nuovo*—chefly, pricey, wear Prada), then add on data provided by neighborhood, décor (or lack of), and prices, and instinctively know if the place will be full of *people like us*. The very best places can pitch themselves with such nuance, they manage to attract not just one type, but many different sorts who are united by more subtle traits than the size of their paychecks and what's on their backs.

Wódka, naturally, was one of those. At first, it had an especially wide range because Jan was incapable of charging his friends for more than a fraction of what they'd consumed. In our twenties, we— I moved in a small herd—frequented mostly Indian places, because the bastardized Bangladeshi curry is the real national dish of England and is extremely good, and is a bargain. Italian and Greek food also got a look in (and I'm just going to detour here to point out the miraculous fact that the very same places we haunted twenty years ago—The Marathon, an appalling after-hours Greek in Chalk Farm; Pollo, a Soho Italian cafe, and nearby Bar Italia—are *still occupying* center stage for today's young London hard-living style-snobs, even though they can now choose from forty billion new options. I find that very comforting). So, Wódka was beyond my budget, but welcomed me anyway, plus many other friends of Jan's, and of mine—carpenters, lawyers, music promoters, actors, journalists, unemployed drummers—and of his sister, Marysia, who was a top fashion PR at the time and had hundreds of loud, beautiful, intimidating friends. Most evenings ended in the morning with more shots of Zubrówka, and dancing on the tables. I do not exaggerate.

I continued to be an irregular regular at Wódka because over the years I bounced constantly back and forth across the Atlantic— I lose count of the leaving parties I had there. I'd taken to writing guidebooks—at first just London, then also New York. This was great, because I was obliged to eat at all restaurants, and this was awful, because I was obliged to eat at all restaurants. (Plus, the only way to make a decent living out of guidebooks is to write, update, and contribute to several at once. Or, preferably, to own the company.) Okay, yes, yes, it is fabulous to have carte blanche, even if you're scrambling for freelance magazine reviewing assignments to pay the restaurant checks (most guidebooks don't) and relying on the largess of strangers—AKA restaurant PRs and unpromising dates—to fund your more extravagant forays. (Truth in travel? Oh, you'd be surprised at how brittle that pious little phrase can be.) But the problem was, while I was eating around these two metropolises—for several years—I craved, more than ever, a restaurant to call home.

In London, it was easy: I'd simply eat where I had to, then go to Wódka for a nightcap. But in New York, I hadn't even found my home base or my friend base, let alone my home restaurant base. Then in 1992, I lucked into an apartment on the corner of Elizabeth and Spring Streets, one of those New York permanently rent-controlled sublets that weld you to the spot forever because the deal's unrepeatable, and so I stayed. It wasn't hard. Manhattan had inspired love at first sight anyway, and had been growing on me ever since. After all, it has 18,000 restaurants. And it wasn't just the quantity, it was the fact that here, unlike anywhere else I knew, people *lived* in restaurants. Oh sure, there are café cultures from Berlin to Barcelona, but here was a real *restaurant* culture, where everyone claimed not merely a basic home restaurant, but a whole repertoire: one for everyday breakfast; one for weekend brunch; one for refuge from the studio apartment; a few for chef worship; for breakups; for first dates; anniversaries; cocktails; extreme hunger; burgers; diets; and so on. Oh, and when they weren't sitting in a restaurant, they were eating there anyway, because every place delivered. And everyone, but everyone, had fierce opinions and the desire to disseminate them. Heaven. Except for the one thing: I lacked a place of my own.

I ate around and eavesdropped promiscuously. I learned a lot about the city. My own neighborhood bordered everything while itself lying low, and confused. Under my (second-floor) kitchen the goodfellas of the Society of St. Joseph's sat on metal chairs, monitoring; next to them were two rival Chinese laundries; beneath my living room was a bodega that got real busy around 2:00 A.M. and was eventually closed by the NYPD narcotics division; across from that was a shop called, appropriately, Just Shades. The nearest restaurants were six blocks away, across Broadway and into SoHo, or down a bit into Little Italy, for soggy linguine and tourists.

Then, around 1995, Elizabeth Street embarked on a dramatic metamorphosis. Slowly at first, then faster than the eye could see, not a *Vogue* went by without mentioning the cunning little boutiques, and the streets grew thick with models. Soon, my secret neighborhood was "Nolita" (North of Little Italy, but everyone knows that now) and there were loads of restaurants. There was Cafe Gitane for focaccia sandwiches and posing with a cigarette; the Kitchen Club for Dutch-Japanese food from an ex-performance artist; Bistrot Margot for *tarte aux blettes* in French; Lombardi's for fabulous brick-oven pizza; MeKong for Vietnamese with attitude; the divey, homey M&R Bar; and the pricey, fancy Rialto. I went to them all, and they were good, but they weren't home.

There was one more place, though. It had opened quietly, a little away from the pack on Cleveland Place. It looked promising with its front wall of glass that folded back in summer, its ocher walls, white-papered tables, and old bentwood chairs. I walked in; it was deserted. I kept walking through and—*woosh!*—like Alice in *Through the Looking Glass*, I found myself in a lush garden. It was paved in brick and shaded by grapevines; around the edges were beds of tomato plants and herbs. A street sign read Rue Rude. Everywhere you looked were frogs: stone ones, green plastic ones, marionette ones, votive candleholder ones. There was a pleasant murmur and titter and clatter from several tables, all crowded with handsome bistro food. Everyone looked happy. I'm sure I did. My food memory is normally photographic (or whatever the taste version is), but I'm not sure what I ate that day, because every dish on Le Jardin's menu has become as familiar as my own cooking. I probably had Gerard's terrine for a start. Then, his *bouillabaisse? Coq au vin? Cassoulet?* Or something with fries, like the *onglet?* Or something light: tuna tartare? Hell, I don't know; it was all good.

Le Jardin wasn't an instant home because, though I loved it, it didn't know me. Or, I should say, Gerard Maurice didn't. A tall, crinkly-eyed Breton of intermittent portliness—depending on whether he was on the wine or the wagon—Gerard turned out, on closer acquaintance, to be the ideal restaurateur, to the manner born. As a chef, he knew what he cooked and he cooked it; as a host, he knew whom he liked and you knew it. Luckily for the restaurant, he had catholic tastes in people, and luckily for me, a particular soft spot for writers. Suddenly I found the "where shall we go" question easy to answer (I was no longer obliged to eat everywhere). Le Jardin was good for all occasions: dates, birthdays, business talks, family visits, tête-à-têtes, big groups. In summer, the garden was heaven; in winter, the coziest tables in the city were inside. My attachment grew so strong, I thought I may as well make it formal, and I started reserving a weekly Wednesday table for twelve in the garden. It was part dinner party, part salon, part matchmaking arena, part networking op, with every week a different cast. Gerard beamed—there were lots of writers—and sent out bottles of Gaillac. One Wednesday was my birthday. Gerard sent out Champagne, and a cake made by his baker friends at Ceci-Cela, with a marzipan me on top, in boxing gloves (that too is another story). Then he invited me to the Vendange.

Every year, on the first Sunday in October, Le Jardin participated in the noble rite of *vignerons* throughout France and held a
fête for the successful harvest of the grapes—the difference here
being that the guests would actually perform the harvest at the party,
and tread the grapes for the annual bottle (just the one) of Le Jardin
appellation. By this time—almost a year had passed—I knew any
bash of Gerard's was bound to be unmissable, but this turned out
to be an all time legendary do. The garden was denuded of tables,
except for the ones staggering under food loads: vast vats with three
kinds of cassoulet; a giant terrine; duck liver mousse; entire wheels
of cheeses; trays and trays of Ceci Cela's petits fours; and a tower-
ing, glittering *croquembouche*. We ate; we drank; we picked the
grapes—augmented by bunches from the Korean deli attached by
clothespins—to the accompaniment of an accordionist in striped
sweater and beret; we encouraged the designated grape-treading
damsel in her labors with raucous French song.

But my favorite part of all was the company. Since I knew only
Gerard, I'd made him introduce me to someone, and that someone and his fiancée and I got on so famously that I was invited to
their regular table at Le Jardin—a monthly lunchtime one of around
half a dozen writers. Well, this group—like this restaurant we'd all
chosen—fit me perfectly. There ensued seven years (and counting) of terrine and *onglet* and *cassoulet;* Gerard's ripe and often incomprehensibly Franglais stories; vicissitudes in all our lives; books
published; jobs left; relationships ended; relationships begun. These
people became, separately and together, just about my best friends.
One of them took me to the party where I met my husband—
fortune directly attributable to the good karma of the right restaurant. Or, as Gerard once put it—"Ah, yes. Time is the clue and
everything go to be good." I'm not sure what it means either.

eating africa

{ F A I T H   A D I E L E }

THE VILLAGERS LOOK at my sister and me and start to cry. Time and again it happens. We are strolling down a village road at dusk, hand in hand, companionably quiet, our feet red with dust, and some village woman stops pounding yam in mid-thrust, the heavy wooden pestle suspended above her head, and drops her jaw.

"*Chineke*," she gasps, looking from Adanna to me to the sky, where *Chineke* resides. "Can she be *mmuo?*"

Our hands fly to our mouths at the suggestion—me, a ghostly ancestral spirit reappeared from the land of the dead—and Adanna burbles with laughter. The truth is almost equally fantastic. At age twenty-six, an unknown half-sister with a face much like hers has appeared from across the sea, from America.

We laugh, hurrying down the path before the others can hear the woman's frantic shouts to "Come see—o!" and run out of the house, wiping their hands on their bright, Dutch-printed *wrappas,* ululating like a wedding party: *"Ul la la la la la!"*

Or we are lounging in the embrace of the giant *achee* tree ("We dry the leaves for soup!" my stepmother Auntie Grace crows, but I am more impressed by the roots, arcing out of the ground higher than a man), waiting for the afternoon heat to pass. As we gnaw on the bright mango pits I can't get enough of, some distant-distant cousin will drive by in a battered Peugeot belching a halo of sour diesel and smack his long pink palm against his inky forehead.

"Oh ho!" he shouts, nearly piloting the vehicle into the ditch, a move my father is famous for. "Are there suddenly two Adannas now?"

I accept the village's attention as I have always accepted tribute, with the tight, unspoken greed of the addict, the flex in the heart muscle, the warmth spreading through the bloodstream. This time it is not about being female, but the hunger, the expectation, is still the same—to see myself conceived, given shape, in the mirror of another's eyes.

I accept these laughing and sobbing women, these nearly smashed cars, as confirmation that I belong in this stranger-family. Yes, I may be the American, absent for twenty-six years, raised in the Land of Flavorless Chicken, Home to Frankenstein Tomatoes, a Nation of Pets Who Eat Small, Dry Stones. But my face is the password, the key unlocking the door to family.

My new sister tends to be shy in the morning, as if each day, after the deep forgetfulness of night, she needs to accustom herself to the idea of me. Whereas I've had twenty-six years of being the only girl, she's only had twelve. Long before I drag myself out of heavy African sleep, I dream her beneath my window, pacing the courtyard, begging the others to wake me.

"Biko, I beg—o," her voice peals, "go and call Auntie." She is too young to claim the privilege of waking me, fourteen years her senior and American to boot.

The others laugh and go about their chores, their refusals receding from the clear bell of her voice. No one wants to be the one to wake the American. I am the only one allowed to sleep through my father's 4:00 A.M. prayer services, the one permitted to dine in pajamas.

I suspect my special status is a combination of factors: chauvinism—the commonly-held belief that anyone from America is more delicate than undiluted African stock; guilt—given that I've been fatherless for twenty-six years, the least he can do is let me sleep late; fear—who knows, after all, what I am capable of, if angered? I'm twenty-six years a stranger. Does anyone really want to take me, the hungry houseguest, on?

Morning in Igboland arrives with a variety of sounds and smells: First the mournful, pre-dawn dirges learned from missionaries, the same nuns who hung a heavy copper bell on my father's arm to stop him from using his left hand. Then the rustle of family members returning to the morning's tasks, the splash of water rising from the well, the sizzle as palm oil heats up, releasing its nut-musk scent, the plop of thick slices of *ji* dropping into a water-swollen pot. This is true yam—not the sweet, orange-yellow, New World pretender that stole its African name. This white-fleshed tuber balances on the head, thick and dark as firewood, and claims responsibility for the high twin birthrate.

I dream the glottal murmur of Igbo, thick and restful to my untrained ears. Someone picking fruit, the crack of stick against trunk, the rustle of leaves resisting the harvest, accompanied by the blooming floral bouquet of pawpaw and citrus and mango. The bleat of the goats that follow me everywhere from a careful distance. They wait around the corners of the house for me like a gang of bearded thugs, smelling my difference.

When the air thickens, burning mist off the tangled greenery, my body shifts in sleep, positions itself to process Africa swirling through the open window. Bugs purr steadily like the generator out back. I open my eyes to a dim room, a Welcome! banner strung across the wall.

By the time I emerge, Adanna has placed a bucket of cool water for my shower in the east bathroom and a basket of fresh-peeled green oranges on the hall table. She is nowhere to be seen.

Bringing Adanna out into the open is like taming one of the family goats. *Nwaiyo bu ije*, as the Igbo say: *Slow is the journey.* After my shower, I sit alone at the table, ignoring the perfect rectangles of bread with brands named Jubilee, Our Lord's, Love, and Dollar that taste much like bread sent on a ship from Britain might taste. Like a con man playing the shell game, I pop the lids off and on a breakfast bounty: golden disks of fried plantain, white porous slabs of yam, pinkish black-eyed peas, and a stew of sunny egg swirled into rich tomato sauce that reminds me of the one African dish my Scandinavian-American mother learned before my father left. "Come watch," she would instruct, parking me on a kitchen stool so I could see her wooden spoon churning peanut butter into tomato sauce—a vivid, oily spiral of red and brown. "Groundnut stew. This is your father's people's food." I would hold my breath, my dislike of peanut butter battling my hunger for a world beyond the Scandinavian palate of black pepper and dill.

When I was six, my mother had reconciled with her parents and moved us to their farm. There I had grown up like any other Scandinavian girl, picking out bones from layers of over-cooked salmon and potatoes, slipping slippery spoonfuls of prune *marjapuuro* to the cat beneath the dinner table, praying for spice. "Why do you think I left in the first place?" my mother muttered.

Now I hover between American coffee and British tea, the two colonizers battling it out on my father's kitchen table, though I sus-pect the presence of the upstart American is a recent addition in my honor. The instant I take my first sip, Adanna tiptoes into the hallway behind me, and positions herself behind the latticework of the courtyard wall.

I ignore her, immersing myself in the ritual of breakfast. It has always been my favorite meal, particularly now that lunch and dinner are mountains of impenetrable starch—cassava paste or cornmeal mush or pounded yam—meant to be swallowed with only the aid of soup ("Don't chew!" everyone shouts helpfully as I hack and wheeze). Once I am fully engaged, she speaks: "Auntie, good morning!"

"Mm-hmh!" I snort, almost like a real Igbo elder, acknowledging her greeting but taking care not to turn from the table. *Slow is the journey.* I don't want to startle her. I dip fist-sized chunks of *ji* into stew and gnaw away, wondering where the fabled African spice that launched ships is.

My mother once told me that giving birth to me was like becoming immortal. She laughed at my suggestion that pregnancy cost her her youth, despite the facts that her father threw her out for having a fatherless black child and she was forced to leave college and move into the projects. I remember spending all day on the crosstown bus, then staggering off, laden with bags of greasy, government-surplus cheese and strange dried grains like bulgur she had no idea how to prepare. Our apartment swelled with international students who brought plates of vegetable curry in exchange for groundnut stew. I didn't know we were poor, but I could taste the threat of it—a chalky flavor like scorched kidney beans. For years I refused to eat anything brown, anything that came in bulk.

"No, becoming a mother was not the end but the beginning." My mother had smiled. "After you were born, I wasn't afraid of death anymore. There was only peace, the self enduring through time."

Finally I understand. Every morning I see Adanna is like giving birth: The moment of stunned joy, then recognition. Me, an only child, suddenly after twenty-six years transformed into twins.

There we are. The strength of what I feel for this stranger startles me. It is so big and new that I carry it like a farmer carries a bellyful of starch to his fields.

I turn quickly and spy my sister in profile, her dark, shining eyes peeking through the open grille of the wall. Caught, she chuckles low in her throat.

"Adanna," I call her, extending the near-ritual invitation like any good African, though I know that she must have eaten hours ago. "Come and eat!"

"Thank you," she sings, dancing in from the courtyard, shaking her head, one hand behind her back. Later, after my breakfast, she will creep into my room with a book, a game, an offering of fruit. She hovers inside the doorway, blocking the sun. Adanna in silhouette.

"Come!" I gesture that she should join me at the table. The insistent Nigerian elder.

She shakes her head, grinning, and then turns serious. "There are some people here to see you," she announces.

I panic at the thought. "What people?"

"People," she answers heavily, placing a finger across the soft petals of her mouth and squishing her nose. She pouts. Visitors require action from us both. She gestures towards the courtyard, where voices can be heard exchanging the traditional *Ngwa* greeting.

Each day has brought an endless stream of relatives from all parts of Igboland. The earliest to arrive are old women bent from having hiked kilometers through the forest from villages they left before dawn. A cousin cooking outside over the big, black cauldron usually spots them coming down the road and rouses the household.

My father and Auntie Grace run out to meet them. *"Da!"* they cry. Auntie! "We were coming to you! How could you walk all this way—o? Why didn't you send a boy to call us to fetch you?" Ushering the staggering sister or aunt or cousin or in-law into the dining room, they call for the cousins to bring food and kolanut.

As the woman sinks into a chair, she is already protesting that she must leave to get back to her fields. "I just had to see if it was true," she says. "I hear that our long-lost daughter has returned from overseas. I have come to see with my own eyes."

These same eyes regard my father steadily. The Igbo phrase for considering new ideas is literally to chew words; accepting them is swallowing. As the trays of soup arrive, my new relative looks far from hungry.

After a while I am summoned. She starts ululating and clapping as soon as she sees me. *"Nno, Nno!"* Welcome! She then faces upward. *"Chineke,* can this be true? Thanks be for our long-lost daughter who has found her way back home to us!" She comes back to me, fingers working her head-tie, which has become loosened in all the excitement. "And your dear mother, is she well?"

"Yes, *Da,* thank you."

She laughs, turning to my father, and asks him to explain this miracle all over again. This twenty-six-year-old birth.

Soon we're huddled in the courtyard, bent over the steaming cauldron, Auntie Grace emerging from the storerooms to show me the family's stock of salt fish, oil bean, and cocoyam, my new Auntie pinching *okazie, achee,* and bitter leaf beneath my nose, a cousin handing me a pestle with a grin and a handful of dried shrimp and melon seeds, everyone concerned with soup lessons for the American.

I see that what Adanna has been holding behind her back is a fresh-picked mango, its ends blushing pink. I can smell the florid, musky scent from where I sit at the table, awaiting new family. Most likely she spent the time I was lying in bed selecting the perfect mango to share with me. The fat, reddish-green fruit is a prize from the tree planted on the occasion of her birth.

Her natal tree stands in the back corner of the compound next to our brothers' palm and breadfruit trees. What about me? I wonder if my father stumbled out into a cold Canadian spring the morning he got word of my birth and chipped a hole in the hard ground with a spoon till it bent. Did he tell anyone, "I'm a father today!" though the child was born thousands of miles away, in western America, and he would not see her for nearly three decades? Did he mark the day alone on the half-frozen earth of some northern country where nothing grows? Did he commemorate the day at all?

After eleven years spent studying in the West, he was no doubt too poor to buy a tree to plant. His occasional windfall made its way in ten-dollar increments to my mother for groceries or books. Perhaps he transplanted a daffodil, my birthday flower, stolen from the campus flower beds; perhaps he poured some beer as libation to the ancestors across the sea and broke a piece of *oji,* kolanut, purchased from the local bodega.

The sharing of kolanut is the traditional Igbo welcome. The first thing my father did when I stepped foot inside his house was to pray over a tray of pink and white kolanut curled tight like tiny fetuses. "Take them, take them," Auntie Grace urged, tucking the caffeine-rich *oji* and its traditional accompaniments—round eggplant called "garden egg" and large spicy pepper known as "alligator pepper"—into my pockets. "You can enjoy them later." I smiled at the irony. Kolanut tastes unbearably bitter—too bitter for most Westerners—but it settles the stomach, and afterwards, I discovered, water tastes incredibly sweet.

I have yet to ask modern, educated Auntie Grace whether or not she buried my siblings' umbilical cords and afterbirth beneath the roots of their natal trees. If she did, it must be comforting to know under which tree one's origin rests, to be able to stand on one's ancestral homeland and feel oneself growing beneath. How is it to taste the fruit of a tree nursed on the same nutrients that gave one life?

No wonder the Igbo always return to the village to build a house in which to grow old. How far, across how many oceans, can we stray before the goddess of the earth calls us back? We return, with all our wealth and degrees, chanting our titles, to sit in the spot where our father's father's father sat, and watch the sun go down. Or, we return, unspoken words clogging our throats, hungry for something. I imagine that death comes as not so great a shock, and that burial is no more than a return to the familiar network of roots that have held one close since birth.

And me, how do I begin to belong some place I have not been planted?

As the Igbo like to name their children, *Ibuadinma*: Two together ensure the good. *Ofu ife adaraii*: One thing does not walk alone. *Som'di bu ajo afa*: I-am-alone is a bad name.

"Come!" I gesture again to my sister that she should bring her mango and join me at the table.

And this time she does.

how to fry an egg

{ CHRISTINE BASHAM }

"**F**INISH YOUR PEAS (or tuna patties, or Salisbury steak). There are children starving in Asia."

Every night, it seemed, I heard this refrain as I sat in the dining room and poked at my food while my father glared at me. My offers to mail the peas to Cambodia made no difference. I should be grateful for the food, for the effort.

And then at twenty-one, blushing bride and newly hired English teacher, I moved to Thailand. My husband and I quit our jobs in America, sold almost all we owned, and said goodbye to our crying families at the airport. As the plane left D.C., I felt drained of energy—and of just about everything else. We spent the next twenty-seven hours in planes and airports—from home to the West Coast, from Seattle to Japan, from Tokyo to Bangkok. At Bangkok's Don Muang International Airport we disembarked, and were immediately overwhelmed by the contrasts. The March air stuck to us, heavy and damp.

Everyone seemed to know exactly where to go, except for the two of us. And at five-foot-three, for the first time in my life, I was tall.

❖

WE SPENT THE night in a hotel, and awoke refreshed and amazed. There were palm trees outside our window, and bottles of water in the bathroom. Cowed by all I'd heard about the dirty Thai tap water, I used the bottled to brush my teeth.

Before the last leg of our trip, we ate breakfast in the hotel restaurant: a thoroughly American breakfast of eggs, sausage, toast, marmalade, coffee, and tea. The waiter took a few seconds to show me the proper way to eat papaya: glistening with a fresh squeeze of lime. It instantly became one of my favorite foods.

We boarded the plane to Chiang Mai, an hour's flight north of Bangkok, in the mountains near Burma. From the plane, everything was the deep, jade green of rice paddies, or the dusty brown of roads and teak trees. Chiang Mai is Thailand's second largest city, but it is a distant second. Hardly a city at all. Back then it was quiet, and slow, and far from cosmopolitan. It was the land of all those starving children my parents told me about, or so I expected.

And yes, in parts of Thailand there were children surviving on little more than rice and fish sauce. That's not what I saw, though. Day after day, meal after meal, Thailand offered luscious, vibrant abundance. Every bite was full of flavor—chilies and garlic, sugar and salt, peanuts and coconut. Just delicious, and amazingly good. After a while, the strange Thai flavors became familiar to me— not ordinary, by any means, but comforting and homey.

After a hard day's work, I'd walk the mile or so to the soup vendor for a bowl filled with plump won tons and collard greens. On chilly December mornings, I'd buy little sugared doughnuts and hot, sweet soy milk from a cart on the side of the road, and walk back home with my body warm and my soul satisfied.

There was food everywhere. Even the post office parking lot had a pickle vendor, selling plums and olives and guava to pucker my mouth, and a fruit man who would tuck a little packet of salt, sugar, and peppers in with my jicama slices or spears of pineapple. At lunch, I'd eat in the school cafeteria. Maybe a curry, with tender bits of beef and plump green eggplants the size of apricots. Fried rice or noodle soup with fish balls or slices of pork and a few floating leaves of marijuana. I'd sit at the table with my students and follow their lead, adding a little chili, a little fish sauce, some vinegar, and sugar from the condiment rack at the table. We'd eat, and suck the spiciness off our lips and teeth on the way back to class. The peppers, tiny and bright little shards of heat, would burn my gums and wake me up for the second half of the day.

At home, on the weekends, I tried to learn to cook fried rice. It sounded so simple, and the cooks in the cafeteria whipped it up so easily, but I failed, and failed again. For months, I'd push my gluey mass of rice and vegetables into the garbage bag, and send my husband hiking on a path through the palm trees to the bus station, home of my favorite stir-fried vegetables. When I wrote home that I loved carry-out from the bus station, my mother clearly imagined me surviving on crumpled packages of peanut butter crackers and stale coffee. What no one back home could understand was how wonderful every single Thai meal really was. From a simple snack to an elaborate banquet, everything was made with the freshest ingredients and a commitment to good food so elemental to the Thai culture that it seemed, to me, almost automatic. It was easy for the Thai to make my mouth water with even their most ordinary dishes. And seeing that ease—the confidence bred of thousands of generations of Thai cooks—made me more than hungry. It made me envious.

After all, in America, I was a good cook. I could bake my own bread, roast a juicy turkey, sauté and fritter and soufflé and simmer with the best of them. Here in Thailand, however, I was a culinary flop. No matter how I tried, I couldn't duplicate the foods I encountered at a friend's house, or even at the grimiest roadside stand. The recipes in women's magazines left me stumped and hungry and walking to the closest restaurant for lunch. I was a missionary—sent to bring enlightenment to the people of Thailand. But in the kitchen, as in so many areas of life, I learned more from the Thai than I ever taught them. Frustrated, humbled, and eager to learn any way I could, I gave up my arrogance, gave up trying to teach myself how to cook. I turned to the women I knew, instead, hoping to learn from them the way I learned to cook American food in my mother's kitchen: by watching a master at work.

Sunan and Noy and Bouy were the perfect teachers. Each had her specialty and individual style but collectively they adopted me as their silly, incompetent American friend. They were determined to teach me to cook. Like a great cook, a proper cook. Like a Thai. How could I pass it up? I shed my American confidence and slowly learned to watch, imitating their every move in desperate hope that their abilities would somehow rub off. Sunan, pampered and lovely, only cooked when she felt like it. She made beautiful dishes, or nothing at all. For her, cooking was a diversion—not the least bit important. If she happened to hang around after a Bible study and saw me butchering a meal, she'd step in and fix things, just so no one would have to eat my cooking.

"You peel vegetables just like the *farang* in the movies," said Sunan. Who would have thought there was a "way" to peel vegetables? Quickly, I learned that just about everything I did was distinctly American. I cut my long hair short when I was pregnant. I wasted my money on a large apartment, instead of investing in gold. I ate cheeseburgers and buttered toast until the smell oozed out of my pores, like every other white person. A little movie star, a little stupidity, blended together. Predictable, and *farang*. Foreign.

Sunan found me completely frustrating. How could I take a perfectly good orange and peel it (Peel it! Completely! With my bare
hand!) and then expect to serve it to someone? Disgusting. And
completely unimaginative. She gently took my next orange and
scored the peel. With the tip of her blade, she lifted the sections back
to form a sunburst, the only respectable presentation for an orange.
"Didn't you learn this in grade four? Didn't you pay attention?" She
shook her head at my limp explanation that American schools don't
teach fruit carving, or crochet, or flower arranging. She was simply unwilling to believe that American children didn't learn these
practical skills. Standing behind her, craning my neck to follow her
every move, I couldn't believe it, either. If I could cook like a Thai,
and make every meal sparkle like a case of beautiful jewels, I'd gladly
forget fractions and adverbs and the Louisiana Purchase.

Another day, Sunan noted my inferior egg-frying skills. *This,*
I thought, *is a solution looking for a problem. Any idiot can fry an egg.*
Sunan wouldn't stand another minute watching me torture those
poor eggs, a fixture of almost every Thai meal.

"Fine," I said, more than a little tired of being taught all the
time. *"Show* me how your egg is any different than mine. An egg
is an egg."

Sunan could be a real pain in the neck.

⁘

IT'S BEEN TWELVE years since the day she nudged me away from
the propane stove and taught me to fry an egg the right way—
the Thai way. A puddle of peanut oil in a hot pan, and the egg
goes in. Nudge the edges together, a bright yellow eye. Let the top
of the egg steam under the pan lid.

The edges came out crispy and light, the yolk high and creamy
and rich. Perfect. I was completely outclassed. I have not made a
fried egg any other way in more than a decade. And when someone

tries to slip me something "over easy," I nudge them away from the stove and show them the right way to fry an egg. A pain in the neck she may have been, but Sunan could also be absolutely right.

Where Sunan ordered, Bouy laughed. Hand in hand, she walked me through the markets to buy meat and vegetables and little desserts steaming in banana leaves. We'd tie bundles of ingredients to her motorbike and giggle as we teetered home, swerving under our load. Bouy loved food, loved the markets, and loved sharing it all with me. She never pushed me to try the cricket dip or the chicken blood sausages, but she always pointed them out to me. "If you were from my village, we'd eat that together. Since we're in the city, let's have this nice fish, instead." For Bouy, food was nutrition, and ambition, and self-expression, all in one. We understood each other: a pair of foodies far from home, joined by cooking and the men in our lives—her boyfriend was a student in my husband's computer programming classes.

Teaching me her ways of cooking was an adventure for Bouy, too. Every ingredient, every recipe, was worth thinking over and savoring. She taught me to pick through the green beans, not just buy off the top of the pile. She took me to her favorite restaurant, Flying Flag Noodles, where we ate noodle soup so spicy she'd laugh, "Oh, I forget my own address!" She showed me a vegetarian restaurant where I could eat for less than a dime. One afternoon, Bouy came from the market with armloads of food. "I'm making my specialty," she beamed. "It's exotic. From a magazine."

One by one, the ingredients went into the pot. Beef. Broth. Salt. Pepper. Potatoes. Onions. Tomatoes. Her exotic recipe and my mother's easy weeknight beef stew were one and the same. Exotic or homey, I tasted friendship and kindness and patience and love. "Is it right, then?" she asked. And it was. Perfect.

Noy had no time for any of that. Student by day, dairy delivery cyclist by night, and then her husband wanted her to cook, too? Hah! Maybe, *maybe* once a month Noy would pull out all the stops and feed her friends a banquet. We'd spread newspapers on the floor and she would bring us plate after plate of food. *Kai luk keuy. Pak tod. Som tum. Gai yang.* And *tom yum goong* so spicy, so irresistible, that it put my husband in the hospital with a burned, swollen throat. He didn't eat for nearly a week.

When Mike came home, Noy brought him more of her now–infamously spicy shrimp soup. From then on, whenever someone else's cooking earned a compliment, Noy would say "Sure, but would you eat it until you had to be *hospitalized?* Now *that's* good food." Most days, though, Noy and her husband ate simply. Ramen noodles, doctored up with some sweet sausage or shredded pork, with shredded vegetables and a poached egg floating in the soup. Quick and easy and cheap, and still much better than any of the things I would have made. But Noy didn't want to teach me. Anything I learned from her, I had to pick up on my own, dodging her elbows and staying out of the way so she could get it all on the table and be done with it.

⁙

WE'VE BEEN STATESIDE for nearly a decade now. Friends come by the house to learn how to cook Thai food from me. I show them what I know, which is always just enough to make me homesick for Thailand. I cook snakehead fish for the company potluck, and sticky rice with mango for the preschoolers. I can steam a fish, or grill a chicken, or fry a pork chop the only proper way—the Thai way. I make fried rice, nowhere near as good as what I ate in Chiang Mai, but good enough. I can fry an egg.

These days, Thailand is mostly a memory. I'm busy making peanut butter sandwiches and chocolate chip cookies and mashed potatoes and such, slapdash American food that fills one's stomach but never really satisfies me any more. As much as I miss it, we'll never return to Chiang Mai. We're settled here, and raising my parents' only grandchildren. I never make my kids eat every last pea. But when I make a little Thai food, the stir fries and curries and soups and salads that I discovered with Noy and Bouy and Sunan, I pull out all the stops. I spend the day squatting in the kitchen, chopping vegetables on a pile of newspapers or crushing peppers and garlic with a mortar and pestle. I open the windows wide, to let the smell of fish sauce out of the kitchen. I put on old Thai pop music and dance.

Yum Pla Dook Foo (Catfish Salad) is my latest achievement. Without Sunan and Bouy and Noy around, I resorted to the Internet for a recipe.

❖

OIL A BAKING sheet, and cover it with catfish fillets. When I can, I use the kind still attached to the skin. If I can't find that, any fresh catfish fillet will do—tilapia, too. Bake the fillets until they're cooked—a little dry and flaky. Remove them from the oven, and let them cool while the oil heats up, to deep fry. Use a fork to separate the fish into bite-sized pieces. If the fillets have skin, scratch a little with the fork so the fish can fluff up, but leave it attached. Deep-fry the pieces, and drain them. Add paper-thin slices of onion, chilies, scallions, and mint. Sprinkle on some sugar, lime juice, and fish sauce, and tiny minced pieces of garlic. Taste it for balance, just sweet and sour and salty and spicy enough to be perfect. If I'd received a decent elementary education, and paid attention, I'd serve it garnished with a tomato skin rosette and some scallion and chili curls. I know my limits, though. A few lettuce leaves and cucumber slices are just fine.

When I finally set it all on the table, tired but victorious, I can't help but compare myself to those three women. I still feel clumsy, and ignorant, and foreign. Still *farang*, even back in America. But

I'm also still learning, and watching, and trying to cook. I love to share these beautiful foods (and my grandmother's lasagna and my dad's barbeque sauce) with anyone who's the least bit interested. Not that I could ever really teach it—I want to share because I still remember basking in Sunan's pride in my first perfect egg, running hand-in-hand with Bouy at the vegetable market, and squatting in the kitchen with Noy to throw together a fast and fabulous meal. I want to share with my friends, and with my children, that sense of adventure and Thai reverence for the friendships and food that make life worthwhile. I feed my sons just a little from my own spoon. "Come on. This is good food. Put down that chicken nugget and *eat.*"

it's the region, not the vegan

{ KARA GALL }

Ï AM A FORMER flaming carnivore. I blame it on my dad, whose own carnivorous tendencies reflect his livelihood as a beef farmer in south-central Nebraska. Growing up on the farm, I ate beef for breakfast, lunch, and dinner. I fell asleep to the sound of lowing cattle and woke in the spring to the wafting scent of thawing manure.

Every year, as part of my summer 4-H activities, I participated in the Market Steer Project—choosing two feeder calves from my family's herd in the spring to raise to market weight. I spent my summers fattening two steers and training them to be led by halter rope. Every morning and evening, I lugged two five-gallon buckets of corn out to the corral. My dad's steadfast rule, "They eat before you eat," meant I had to feed the steers before I ate breakfast and supper (in the Midwest the *noontime* meal is called "dinner"). Throughout the summer, my steers gained between four and six hundred pounds. In August, I showed them off at the Fair and Corn Show, often winning first place in the rate-of-gain contest. While some 4-Hers planned to sell their animals at the local, county, or state fairs, or directly to a meat packer, my steers were shipped off to the beef processing plant every October where they were turned into the ground beef, T-bone steaks, and rump roasts that adorned the center of our dining room table. We kept the meat from one animal in our basement freezers and sold sides of beef from the other to my aunts and uncles who lived in more metropolitan areas. My parents put the money from the sales into my college fund. Beef is in my blood.

Even so, these days I consider myself a tentative vegan—one who eats no animal products. My father blames this (along with my tattoos, piercings, dyed hair, and unshaven legs) on the state of California, and has suggested that my eating habits will turn me into a lesbian. Though I personally don't associate my penchant for girls with my eating habits, I won't argue that food and sexuality are intricately intertwined. (And I can advise you, from personal experience, never to prepare anything with habanero peppers on a night you expect any sort of hands-on intimacy with your lover. Though in desperate times, the habanero can be an effective break-up strategy.)

Peppered palms aside, why would a corn-fed, farm-bred Nebraska girl like me choose the hot-'n'-spicy meatless path? Don't get me wrong. I'm no militant vegan. I'm not looking to debate the many moral, spiritual, environmental, and economic benefits of shunning animal products. For when I said "tentative vegan," I meant I have yet to renounce the sausage. I still believe in the power of cheese. Whole milk—especially the kind with the cream plug left on top—makes me shiver with delight. A girl raised in Eustis, Nebraska—the *Sausage Capital* of Nebraska—doesn't dare sever her flesh-eating roots completely. The sausage, known as *wurst* in German, has become an ancestral talisman for my hometown, whose German heritage has been kept alive through customs, foods, and celebrations. The motto of the Wurst Haus, the local grocery store and sausage deli is "You'll love our wurst." I worked there during summers, stuffing sausages. Bratwurst, liverwurst, blood-wurst, Polish: they all hold a hallowed place in the refrigerator of my memory. The venison, beef, and pork used to make the sausage are still purchased from local farmers and hunters. Every year, the chamber of commerce produces a community celebration called Wurst Tag, or "Sausage Day." This celebration, something akin to Oktoberfest, attracts people from all areas of the state who want to binge on German food, beer, and polka dancing. The popula-tion of the town triples and sausage sales soar. The *spätzle*, pret-zels, *runzas*, sauerkraut, red cabbage, plum *kuchen*, German chocolate cake, and Springerle cookies served at the Wurst Tag com-munity dinner were all staples in my childhood diet.

Even so, my homeland taught me something much deeper than sugar, meat, and dairy. If you are bold enough to push my milk curds aside and look beyond my sausage casings, you will discover a pulsing, natural, herbivorous rhythm in the landscape of my youth. In high school, I spent my weekend nights at pasture parties, where groups of teenagers would gather amongst the cattle to party where the county sheriff could not find them. I surrendered my virgin-ity in a cornfield: earth beneath me, stars above, and a rather uncomfortable pickup truck door at my back. Even the state uni-versity's mascot reflects the regional relationship to food; the Uni-versity of Nebraska Cornhuskers have the following of a professional football team.

In the summer, we picked wild plums and blackberries from the bushes and trees that skirted our pastures and boiled the juice with gelatin to make sweet jellies and jams. The food on my family's dinner table had literally swayed in the fields beyond our dining room window. We did not buy frozen meals, TV dinners, or microwave popcorn. Every Sunday night, Dad made flapjacks on the griddle, complete with eggs my sister Rachel and I had gathered from the chicken house. We canned our own vegetables and stored meat from our own cattle in the basement freezers. My family planted a garden every spring—rows of green beans, radishes, tomatoes, sweet corn, lettuce, rhubarb, zucchini, cucumbers, and squash. A little section of our garden was squared off for compost, where lawn clippings, fruit rinds, and manure from the corral fermented to make a rich loam. Rachel and I were given garden chores: We were expected to weed the garden once a week and pick, wash, and snap the green beans every other day. As summer blazed on, my mom spent at least twenty hours a week in the kitchen, canning beans, beets, and rhubarb and stewing tomatoes for the winter. Dozens and dozens of Mason jars filled the storage room in the basement, each labeled on the tin lid to indicate the current year. My sister and I diligently rotated the jars so that the previous years' supply was in front and the more recent canned goods were in the back.

In August, we packaged and froze sweet corn for the winter. It was a family affair. We rose at dawn in order to get most of the work done before the hot sun rose too high in the sky. We set up our shucking stations off the back porch of the house. Dad pulled two huge steel tubs out from the washhouse and set two lawn chairs in front of each tub, each of which measured about two feet in diameter and when filled held over five gallons of water. Dad and Rachel teamed up in front of one tub, while Grandpa and I took the other. With four burlap bags full of sweet corn between us, we competed to see whose team could shuck the most. We each took an ear of corn, ripped off the husk, and pulled the fine cornsilk from the cob. After only a few ears, the moist little yellow tassels were stuck to my arms, legs, and face. The clean ear of corn was placed in the steel tub and the husk was dropped into a wheelbarrow. Grandpa and I were quick—once we hit our groove, we shucked each ear in just two quick strokes. My sister and my dad were not always so productive. If they were getting along they were impossible to beat, but more often than not their shared competitive nature worked against them, and they soon began arguing about the best shucking strategy. Before you knew it, one of them had stomped off angrily, leaving the other cursing with the remainder of the corn. Grandpa and I laughed quietly, assuring each other that our way would prevail. As the sun and the temperature rose, I peeled off layers of clothing, so that by nine o'clock I was down to a tank top and cutoffs and willingly dipping my hands in the frigid well water that filled the washtubs. When the wheelbarrow was full, I ran it over to our horse Streak, who munched on husks all day long. Every half-hour or so, Grandma would come outside to empty the naked ears of corn from our tubs. My mom and grandmother worked together in the kitchen, slicing the corn from the cob and then packaging it in vacuum-packed freezer bags. It was a job I was happy to let them do—I loved being outside where the dog paced between tubs, giving equal time to everyone in the family and occasionally snagging an ear out of the tub and burying it behind the washhouse like a bone.

We saved a couple dozen of the fresh ears to eat from the cob, slathered with butter and salt. Rachel and I tried to poke the little cob holders into the edges so we wouldn't burn our hands, but Dad threw a tizzy fit. "Those things are for city people!" he proclaimed, leaving me to speculate that maybe city people were a bit smarter, if only for not wanting to burn their hands.

Being a city girl myself these days, I can guarantee that we are by no means any smarter than rural bumpkins when it comes to food. City folk have more choices, maybe—where organic is trendy, vegetarian and vegan options top the menus at the local restaurants, and a rich ethnic diversity widens the spectrum of the palate.

When I moved to California over five years ago, I was amazed and overwhelmed by the availability of organic produce and vegetarian cuisine. I fumbled around with new foods—I did not know how to peel garlic; I had only heard tell of avocados in the context of guacamole. I ordered *edamame* at a sushi restaurant once and was shocked to find out they were only soybeans, soybeans like my father grows. What I thought were small twigs in my soup turned out to be rosemary! I didn't know my shiitake from my wasabi. I needed to be taught how to eat mangos, pomegranates, and persimmons. A new world of taste overrode my childhood palate of meat, beans, and potatoes. Hummus, falafel, tabbouleh, salsa—I couldn't get enough. I quickly learned the spicy, delectable joys—and dangers—of cooking with habanero peppers.

But though this exotic new culinary world felt glamorous and dangerously decadent, I became all too aware that preparing a meal was not as simple as heading out to the garden, or down to the basement. Trendy food and family meals do not often go hand in hand. I resented standing in half-hour lines at the grocery store just because I forgot to buy milk for my daughter Lydia's lunchbox. I'd had it with those stupid little Goldfish that get all over the car, in between the couch cushions, and (mysteriously) under the sheets. I was sick of breakfasts on the run. Lydia didn't want to eat persimmon and pomegranates. She scrunched up her nose at avocados and stuck out her tongue at sushi. Forcing her to eat hummus meant anything from an hour of her crying to her dramatizing a self-induced throwing-up scene. Night after night I begrudged the time I spent in the kitchen trying to prepare a well-balanced, child-friendly meal that ultimately ended with my daughter whining, "I don't like that." When I didn't get home from work until six and bedtime was at eight, I wondered which was more important to my sanity—convenience or health. Whenever I pulled out the pen and notepad to make a weekly menu, I inevitably ended up in the car fifteen minutes later, driving to McDonald's.

Soon thereafter, every time I went to the grocery store, the produce seemed to look at me with shifty eyes. How well did I really know that head of broccoli? How much could I trust the zucchini? And that melon? It sure smelled good, but what did I know of its history? I couldn't picture the furry bovine face behind the ground-beef package stacked in the refrigerated case beside hundreds of other cellophane-wrapped clones. Standing in the grocery aisle, an empty blue plastic basket in my hands, I felt betrayed. I realized I did not know the people who were growing, picking, packing, and shipping the food we were consuming. I missed the freezer full of beef in Mom's basement. I longed for that way of life, where all-natural canned-by-Mom green beans are only a few feet away.

In that moment, it was easy to look back at my childhood on the farm as idyllic, and I indulged in memories of growing up wild in the backcountry of America, living off the land. But the truth is, I loathed the garden chores when I was a kid. I didn't understand then why we had to go through all the work. Why couldn't we just buy our green beans in a can, like my friends' families did? Oh, the irony, that I was now wishing I could grow my own. I cursed the tiny deck of my urban apartment where the most I could grow each summer were a few herbs and tomatoes. I backed away from the foreign broccoli, rolled the alien cantaloupe back into its nest, and wretchedly weaved my way to the checkout stand with nothing but a frozen pizza and a box of jalapeño poppers.

I felt like I was having a bunch of one-night stands with my dinner plate. The intimacy with food that I was craving was not a California thing. It was a Nebraska thing. It had something to do with chicken poop on the bottom of my shoe, the smell of Rocky Mountain Oysters—flame-broiled bull testicles also known as "fries"—on my father's tattered denim work jacket, and the sound of cows happily masticating in the corral beyond my bedroom window. Somewhere between Nebraska and California, I had lost my connection to the source of my food. And it was time to get it back.

I bought a whole foods cookbook and found I actually enjoy eating grains, vegetables, and salads. Green, crunchy, crisp lettuce with tomatoes, nuts, beans, red onions, and avocados. Romaine, buttercrunch, Slobolt, iceberg: a world of lettuce opened up to me. Even more surprisingly, I felt better when I ate this fare. I had more energy. My allergies cleared up. I didn't get sick nearly as often. I actually improved some of my personal relationships because I wasn't using my typical defense mechanisms to deal with stress and vulnerability. I had more time in the evenings because I cooked simple meals with simple ingredients. These days, I take my caffeine in the form of green tea and I spend my Saturday mornings browsing the farmers' market just two blocks from my apartment with my daughter. I've gotten to know the vendors there. I learned that my favorite vendor Valerie's carrots are not certified organic by the USDA because she and her husband are small-scale farmers who cannot afford certification, though they follow organic growing standards. I continue to buy carrots from her because we have developed a relationship, a trust in each other that developed out of many discussions about farmworker advocacy, international corporations' control of agriculture, and the importance of buying locally. As we stroll through the stalls, Lydia manages to talk the strawberry vendors out of a few plump berries and the Taiwanese flower ladies out of stray orchids.

And then we got worms. *Composting* worms. I saved the unused rinds, stalks, and leaves from my fruits and vegetables and fed them to my own little herd of worms in an urban farmgirl sort of way. I use the worms as a measure of what I should or should not put in my body. If they can't easily digest it, I don't eat it. Every spring my daughter and I dry the compost from the worms and use it in our small balcony garden. I am by no means practicing sustainable agriculture, but I am connected.

In the end, my half-baked veganism has more to do with reclaiming this connection to the source of my food than rejecting or romanticizing the lifestyle of my childhood. My relationship to the food I eat is not about whether or not I consume meat or dairy. The point is that on any given day, I am most likely putting food into my body that makes me feel good. And some days I do get a hankerin' for one of the local *taqueria*'s grilled steak tacos. When that happens, I listen to my gut.

farmers' market salad

I never liked salad until I tried this combination of ingredients, all purchased from my local farmers' market. The tastiest part, however, is having a relationship with the folks that grow the vegetables!

Salad

1 head red leaf lettuce

1 head green leaf lettuce

1 bunch baby greens

3 pears, diced

2 cups raisins

2 green peppers, cut into thin strips

1 medium red onion, cut into thin strips

2 avocados, diced

Dressing

½ cup olive oil

⅓ cup balsamic vinegar

1 T. Dijon mustard

1-2 cloves garlic, minced

salt and freshly ground pepper

For dressing, whisk ingredients together. Wash greens carefully, dry completely, and tear into bite-size pieces. Add remaining ingredients and enough dressing to coat. Toss lightly. Serves 4-6.

arroz con humildad

{ L E S L I E   M I L L E R }

There is something rather specifically dismal about a failed rice dish.
—ELIZABETH DAVID

I CAN'T MAKE RICE.

Rice, for God's sake. It's like saying you can't make toast, fry an egg, boil water—which, may I add, is part of making rice.

Long grain white rice. None of the components are even polysyllabic. We're not talking puff pastry here, it shouldn't be that hard. Four lines are devoted to rice preparation in the *Escoffier Cook Book*, barely more in the *Joy*. You don't have to coat it in aspic, wrap it in phyllo, feed it for days like a needy starter—it's not even a *main dish,* not in American culture anyway. Not like in Southeast Asian cuisine, or Japanese *donburi* where rice is featured, lovingly, and a little "cohesion" to the rice is nothing shameful. *Sticky* rice I'm good at. (Since all my rice turns out that way, it's nice when "glutinous" is already in the name.)

That my relationship to sticky rice didn't really come until the ripe age of eighteen seems near ridiculous now that I live in a city famous for Pacific Rim fusion, and in a country that currently can't get enough fresh rolls and *phờ*. But years ago in college, when Southern California still signified vapid Valley girls and vegetarian Venice Beach freaks, I found out that no one from Los Angeles is really vegetarian. Accordingly, I soon discovered that the dorm cafeteria offered the vegetarian nothing inoffensive except corn flakes, cheese sticks, and jicama. I quickly tired of Jicama Five Ways, and decided that cheese sticks really are offensive after all.

I shared my dorm room with Nitta. She was from Waimea, a tiny town on Kauai in Hawaii, and I am from Washington State. The university was full of commuters who went home to San Gabriel, Glendale, West Covina on the weekends—we figured since neither of us could go home for minor holidays the housing board stuck us together. Jeannie Kang lived down the hall.

We used the cafeteria to supply lemons for drinks, and snuck packets of sugar and straws, but for food retreated often to our room, replete with a miniature refrigerator, a rice cooker, and a twenty-pound sack of Calrose rice. We took turns taking the rice cooker to the bathroom at the end of the hall and lovingly filling, rubbing, and rinsing until the water was no longer milky with starch but ran clear, the way Jeannie's mother said you should. Filling the water to the first knuckle of the middle finger as it barely grazed the top of the grains in the pot. Twenty minutes later, after hissing and rumbling and lifting the lid with ladylike burps of starchy steam, the rice cooker would turn itself off. We would wait an additional, agonizing five minutes, to allow the rice to settle, then we'd get out crisp *lavar*, seaweed toasted and brushed with sesame oil and sprinkled with salt. We bought plastic tubs of it at the Korean market but coveted the Ziploc bags–full that Jeannie brought back from LA. Perilla leaves in a fiery red paste, sprinkled with sesame seeds. Bitter burdock root coated in pepper and laced with strips of green onion and ginger. Crisp salted anchovies whose heads popped like Rice Krispies when you bit down on them. And cucumber *kimchi*—my favorite—the explosive fermented odor of which made us enemies of the other residents of the dorm, even the Bengali girls across the hall who made their own delicious, off-smelling concoctions that reminded them of home. On the weekends I'd go to the Korean market with Nitta, restocking our noodle bowls and our sesame oil, fish cake for Nitta, and more *kimchi* for me. "You like *kimchi?*" the owner asked every time, incredulous. When I nodded she'd laugh and touch my blond hair—"So spicy, eh?"

In addition to Jeannie's homemade contributions to our table, Nitta's mom sent care packages of the Japanese-Hawaiian foods Nitta loved and missed, and for a change we splurged on Poi Five Ways and *natto* and stirred an inky, gelatinous concoction of soy and seaweed that looked like Vegemite into our rice with sesame oil and raw egg. My parents sent boxes of Washington apples; they seemed provincial to me, but they were crisp and sweet and we ate them for weeks, a cool foil to the Korean fire. In that room it ceased to matter that Jeannie and Nitta were both seven inches shorter than I, that their thick black hair contrasted with my blond, that Nitta whispered pidgin into the phone to her friends in Hawaii or that Jeannie was harangued by the other Koreans on campus for hanging out with a white girl and for not going to church group. Jeannie gave me a Korean name, Jae-Hee, and we would call each other to dinner like old Korean housewives, *"Jae-heeaaaaaa,"* she would croon. *"Unsookaaaaa,"* I would answer, using her birth name, Un Sook. And then we would eat.

⋰⋱

I CAN'T MAKE rice, and I blame it on my heritage. My people eat potatoes, not rice. They also eat pickled herring with cream, so perhaps I should have learned long ago not to blindly follow my family's culinary culture. Sometimes, I remember, my mother served white rice with her Swedish meatballs instead of the requisite slippery egg noodles, and rice accompanied the classic '60s fad dish (that we still ate in the '80s): "Hawaiian" chicken—swimming in fat, the pineapple too cloying and the peppers bitter and tough from their stint in the oven. But it was rice that came from a box—foolproof; one of mother's little helpers neither acknowledged by grandmothers nor instructive to daughters whose gastronomic pride precludes entertaining the very *idea* of Minute Rice. (I will admit to fond memories of its more Nordic equivalent, though—Potato Buds—a gluey moat that rescued the defenseless green beans from the threat of gravy.)

I blame it on my mother, who did cook wild rice upon occasion—which always seemed to take too long, nearly an hour until it didn't crack the tooth. She served it with pork—roast, not the chops she covered with mushroom soup and simmered in the electric skillet. Wild rice was elegant. Wild rice was served at dinner parties, at the gourmet gatherings my parents rotated with two other couples—dinners of poached fresh salmon fillets and dripping rare hunks of beef encased in rock salt and served with horseradish whipped with cream. I have always thought wild rice pretty, and thought it tastes a bit like dirt—whether minted, fruited, or just tossed with salt, pepper, and butter, I feel it masks the flavor of other dishes with its muddy flavor. I came to find out that it isn't rice at all, but a wild grass native to the United States, and I choose to leave the grasses to bovine gourmands.

Were it that I could make brown rice, instead. Guilted into a whole-foods phase once my *Vegetarian Times* subscription kicked in, the seductively political pages also prompted my first trying quinoa, spelt, and instant brown rice (straight from the box like Mum used to make). I drew the line at Bragg's Liquid Amino Acids, but whatever mysterious process enables instant brown rice to go from box to ready in under ten minutes surprisingly doesn't really do it and its more open, spongy texture a disservice. And with a can of white beans, lots of fresh pepper, some good Parmesan and homemade pesto (from the freezer, from last year's basil), it made many a quick supper for me during college. As I ate I felt, well, healthy, despite the pooling olive oil melting out of the pesto and the addition of consecutive applications of Parmesan.

But white rice can't come from a box. Jasmine, basmati, Texmati —there are whole cookbooks devoted simply to these grains, forming a yawning chasm in my cooking repertoire. These rices, with names like perky toddlers, shame me deeply. They laugh at me from the depths, calling out gently, *fraud*: I am a writer who misuses "affect" and "effect"; I am a computer programmer who uses AOL; I am an athlete who smokes.

It was hard enough to be a vegetarian for fourteen years and nearly cry at the pasta primavera offered as my "choice" in most restaurants. I considered it my mission therefore not to proselytize on the fate of veal calves—there were enough vegans doing that—but instead on the delicate sensibilities of food-loving vegetarians who craved adventure, danger, and flavor on their plates. It made it that much more insulting when, at a dinner party for a couple that claimed vegetarian food uniformly bland and unsatisfying, I once again fell short. The menu: jasmine rice studded with almonds, the perfect accompaniment to complex enchiladas painted with the most carefully constructed *salsa verde*. The filling— *nopales* I scoured Pike Place Market for, fresh corn, pine nuts, and a delicate *panela* that melted into ropey puddles. A quivering cinnamon flan. And the rice. Studded with almonds, yes, but gluey, not delicate. As I served it the spoon mashed the grains until the mass unhappily resembled spotted, beige grits. It is no accident I bought a bottle of Patrón to accompany the dinner; I've learned to pour freely when rice is on the menu. Because of it, up until now, I think my failure has been under wraps.

I can't make rice.

I told my friend Buzzy the same thing when she appointed me head chef of the Mexican dinner we cooked in the plush, modern apartment of the family Lisa Kurtzman nannied for in Barcelona. The family was out and we—Lisa's American "family" of expatriates—were in, loaded with avocados, chilies and beans, rice and cilantro, garlic. None of us was crass enough to have conflated Spanish and Mexican cuisine before we arrived, but after months of *bacalao* and blood sausage and *pan catalana* we just missed what we considered *our* food, the precious *carnitas,* crisp *tortas,* and jeweled *aguas frescas* that came from our neighborhood *taquerias* and taco trucks.

Before the dinner I quizzed Beatríz and Elena from Chicago on their mothers' recipes for rice. They were going dancing instead. They cast eyes at me. A *recipe* for Mexican rice? They didn't have a recipe—they just watched their mothers. Silly *juara.*

"You just make the rice like you make any other rice," Beatríz told me.

"But you add onion before you start, and some garlic but make sure it doesn't burn," added Elena.

"Then you stir the rice in the oil and the onion and the garlic until it's shiny," Beatríz said.

"Then the water or some *caldo* and the tomato chopped up."

"Just one tomato?" I asked.

"You can add more," shrugged Beatríz. *No importa.*

"Then do you change the amount of water or broth that you

add?" I should be able to figure that out, their faces told me. It wasn't that hard—it was just *rice*.

I dutifully chopped the onions and garlic and sautéed them in olive oil. I poured in the rice and allowed it to bathe in the oil, not to the point of toasting but until every grain glistened and had begun to pop. Then water, tomatoes—I measured, I did. I brought it to a boil then lowered the heat and left it to simmer quietly. I never peeked. Instead I rolled out thick, misshapen flour tortillas with a half-empty bottle of Jerez sherry; I crushed garlic and chilies with cilantro and salt and lime, then worked in those perfect avocados.

We were all from LA or at least recent transplants, but universally, these flavors—the bite of the chilies; the intensity of the garlic; the mellow comfort of the soft, soupy beans; the clean soapiness of the fringed cilantro—these flavors signified home to us, three WASPs and two Jews from the Valley. In a week we would watch Los Angeles burn as the riots broke out, the Spaniards clucking their tongues about America's race problems, but for now the nostalgia seemed simple. We drank in that bright kitchen in the Barcelona suburb, so oddly modern and so unlike the propane-heated, antiquated walkups the rest of us shared with Spanish roommates. The wine was from Rioja, but no matter. During that dinner we pretended we weren't situation-poor students with a tenuous grasp of a different Spanish lexicon and slang—*el castellano*—which the Spaniards called "real." We ate tortillas *mexicanas*—not omelets at all but fresh, floury rounds that soaked up salsa, scooped up guacamole, and sopped up the gorgeous beans. And the rice. The flavor was there, the sweet onion rounding out the acidity of the tomatoes from Seville, but the texture: scalded on the bottom, rice pudding on top. No matter that I'd fluffed it with a fork so as not to mash the grains. We ate it anyway—for the memories, to alleviate the heat from the salsa, because of the wine. I blamed the 220-volt stove.

I can't make white rice.

So what to do? Concede and take advantage of the potatoes revival, substitute my starches? Serve parsnip purée or a cheesy polenta? Surely these fads must end, all food fads do—and rice is enduring, 40,000 years of cultivation under its belt. It will stalk me, haunt me, taunting me with my gastronomic ineptitude. My Achilles' heel is formed of a lumpy chain of long-grain rice.

Maybe you don't understand how much this hurts my pride, because I can *cook*. Even rice in some forms. I can make black rice pudding with coconut milk, I roll hospital-corner sushi; I can create elegant, stunning risottos, every grain tender with a delicate firmness just so it keeps its shape—bathed in wine, mushrooms, perhaps kissed by the Moroccan saffron I keep in a paper packet sealed away. My *avgolemeno* soup is light and lemony, both chicken and rice perfectly tender. I have even endeavored to recreate the adzuki beans and rice an old boyfriend used to bring from his Japanese mother's house straight to my own. She would cook pounds of it and freeze it in individual portions to last him until his next trip home to LA. His mother kept feeding him out of duty and love; he brought me her gifts as an offering of calories and culture, a payment for sharing my bed and my kitchen.

Even after I'd begun to grow weary of his company I still ate happily from my freezer until every packet was gone and I was forced to ask for the recipe. He relayed bits and pieces from his mother over the phone. Whether it was a translation issue or whether he suspected it was over, I don't know. Finally, I hunted down the recipe in the biblical *Japanese Cooking: A Simple Art,* soaking the beans and then cooking them until they were just tender. I reserved the liquid and used it to soak the rice overnight, turning it cherry-blossom pink. Then I combined the beans and rice and steamed them, sprinkling with ground sesame seeds and coarse salt. Heaven, no boyfriend required.

But hubris aside, perhaps there's a reason I can't make rice, a reason other than my upbringing, aside from my culture, in spite of my obsession with food. Perhaps this time—this time only—it's not right to blame my mother. For if I am made to endure the fate of Achilles, perhaps it is so my husband can play at being Paris.

My husband used to cook. Holed up in his punk-rock dive with six other smelly, dirty men and last night's beer cans, he used to walk miles to the market to shop, then miles back in the dark in order to cook chickens in clay pots and a Bolognese that took all day, stellar *linguine alle vongole* with fresh thyme, and stewed rabbits in red wine. He tells me. He rarely enters the kitchen in our home except to do dishes, letting me cook because, as he says, I enjoy it. And also, he's admitted, because he's intimidated. And food is clearly something I care more about than he does, more about than many people, I'm sure. I talk about food like some girls talk about shoes; my eyes glaze when we enter the market. I can't food-shop and carry on a conversation at the same time, as he learned long ago. I experiment and cook extravagantly and sometimes fail, but not often. I know my strengths. I bake well. I'm good with fish and with Ethiopian stews and *bisteeya* and hollandaise. I can fill tortelloni and fry feather-light tempura, make airy biscuits and poach an egg. But because of my fairly recent fall from vegetarianism, I'm just now learning to roast meats and make pan sauces and bone chickens—all of those meatless years set me back in a few areas. However, I've noticed that as I attempt to cook more meat, tentatively—poking steaks and touching my hand to tell if they're done, hacking chickens into Frankenpieces because I can't find the joint—my husband has started to pop back into the kitchen. Like most men, he likes to grill, and more than that he likes an even playing field. The science of internal temperatures and resting times is not knowledge special to me, and he can read a cookbook as well as I.

So as I learn to appreciate the feel of another person in the kitchen, I remember that a vulnerable cook is an approachable cook—no one likes a foodie tyrant who slaps your hands off her knives (I don't do that, anymore). Perhaps rice *is* my Achilles' heel—a reminder of vulnerability, a reminder that some of the best moments in the kitchen aren't spent in pursuit of perfection, but in stopping stirring to dance with your partner, in teaching a child the textures and flavors of fruit, or remembering that whisks make great musical instruments and ricers can noodle Play-Doh, and husbands can make a stunning *linguine alle vongole*, if only you let them into the kitchen.

my life among lobsters

{ GRETCHEN VANESSELSTYN }

I DON'T REMEMBER my first taste of lobster, but I can picture it. That phrase, "my first taste of lobster," probably conjures visions of a child in an antique highchair, lace napkin tucked under her chin, a buttery silver spoon bearing an ivory morsel perched at her waiting, ruby lips.

Instead it was a bit of rubbery claw meat, dangled from my father's rough hand, his blue eyes watching to see if I was a true lobsterman's daughter, or a mere landlubber. Legend has it that I laughed, and asked for more, thus cementing my fate, my life among lobsters.

In fact, the truth is somewhere in between. My father, despite his most fervent desires, was a paper executive. Weekdays he would mull new cup designs, sit through meetings about desirable colors and scents for toilet tissue. But on summer nights and weekends, he got to take off his business suit, pull on his cutoffs, his stained T-shirt, and bait-shop hat, and pretend. The corporate world has its rewards: stable hours, decent paycheck, walls to shield you from the cold wind. But you really feel like a provider when you haul up a big load and hear the approving grunts of your fellow fishermen as you carry the pails down the dock. You lay them out on the lawn, just for show, then haul them into the house, where your city-born wife waits knowingly with a pot of boiling water and a pound of butter. Beats bringing home a piece of paper any day.

It was the 1970s, and Long Island Sound was still rich with food: bluefish, fluke, weakfish, stripers. We had twelve pots in the water, which meant three or four lobster dinners a week in the high season. The summer days were long, spent waiting to hear Dad's car pull into the driveway, then waiting again until we were out on the water, salt splashing on my face, wind tangling my hair. We'd cruise up to one of the empty bleach bottles that marked our pots, and the anticipation would build as I watched my father's tan, muscled arms work, pulling up the line and resting the pot on the boat's ledge.

Sometimes we'd bring up a pot teeming with them. Dad sized them, checked for eggs, and tossed the illegals back over the side. The legal ones would go in the boat, and I'd hold my breath as he forced a white, ribbed peg into each claw's hinge so it couldn't snap shut. He'd bait the pot with a chunk of mackerel or bunker, then toss it back over the side.

Sometimes the trap would be empty. Other times a spider crab or two—terrifying creatures with foot-long, eager claws—would wait inside. At the first sight of these sea monsters, I would run to the bow and hide my eyes until Dad said "All clear." But I was never afraid of lobsters.

Back at home, I'd watch them try to fight, try to snap me, each other, anyone. They were angry to be out in the fresh air, but a short, hot bath took care of that. We ate them boiled with melted butter, corn and potatoes on the side.

As a young child I learned to break open lobster shells and extract the meat without using tools, though crackers and picks were always available for guests. Snapping off the tail plates, then pushing my fingers into the niche to force out the meat is a party trick that still impresses, though people now figure that I learned it in cooking school. Rejecting the disgusting green goo in the body cavity, we ate claws and tail first, then sucked the juice from the small, prickly legs.

In summer, we ate from the sea. Huge bluefish steaks, whole roasted striped bass, tiny deep-fried snappers, and whole dynasties of lobsters fed the VanEsselstyns year after year. From May through September, we lived the life of kings, the life of lobstermen.

The rest of the year, Mom got dinner on the table every evening after teaching first-graders all day. Because she attended graduate school at night and raised us two kids, dinner was mostly Hamburger Helper, SPAM, and boxed macaroni and cheese. But it was dinner, and we liked it, and let's forgive those meals for the sin they seem now to be, the heart surgery they brought my father, the thirty extra pounds that stick to my frame no matter what I do. Dad ate strange concoctions: jellied consommé from the Campbell's can, which was kept in the refrigerator, topped with Worcestershire sauce; peanut butter, mayo, and ketchup sandwiches; and hardboiled eggs sliced into a bowl, topped with a generous spoonful of mayo and a sprinkling of cornflakes.

My brother David liked fried eggs, I liked scrambled. For four months, once, I ate only soup, inspired by Russell and Lillian Hoban's *Bread and Jam for Frances*. But all winter we'd bide our time, waiting for that taste of summer, the flavor of salt and sea, of butter and sunshine, that was the first lobster of the year.

❖

WHEN I WAS twenty-five, I met a wonderful man, the funniest person I have ever known. We laughed, we ate Chinese food, we fell in love. And I foresaw a day when I would never eat lobster again. A wedding dress, a canopy. Poached salmon. Roast chicken. My father, a yarmulke sliding off his sun-freckled bald spot. My mother clapping her hands as I teetered above her on a chair, held up by strangers and friends, clinging tight to a handkerchief. On that day, I would trade steamed clams for companionship, oysters for love, lobster for a new way of life.

Danny, my new love, was an Orthodox Jew. I caught him in a rebellious phase, and had great fun introducing him to the pleasures of Saturday morning cartoons, necking in public, and cheeseburgers. When my August birthday rolled around, I took him to Connecticut to meet my family. My dad had sold his lobster pots years before, but we piled into the car and drove to a casual shore restaurant, and sat, looking out onto the Sound. When the waitress came around, my dad said, "Beer, Danny?" He glanced at me and nodded. "We'll have two pitchers of beer, steamers all around, and four lobster dinners," Dad told her. Danny politely passed on the steamers—shellfish, including lobsters, are not kosher.

"It's okay," I whispered to him. "You'll get corn and bread and a potato. I'll eat your lobster."

"No, I'll eat it," he told me. Feeling more than a little guilty, I watched him take his first taste of lobster. "Oh my god. How can anything taste this good?" he asked me. I boiled a lot of lobsters for him over the next year, falling deeper in love with each passing month.

At the Guggenheim Museum gift shop, we found a poster of the Picasso painting *Lobster and Cat.* "That's you," he told me, pointing at the spiky, gray lobster, "and that's me," he said, pointing at the brown cat, its fur on end, terrified. "Thanks a lot," I told him, as he paid for the poster. He hung it on his apartment wall, and I'd look up at it sometimes and realize that he was right. Lobster and Cat. We were about as alike, similarly contentious.

One night, after a few drinks, my brother took me aside. "You guys are getting really serious, huh? If you want, I'll convert with you so you won't be the only Jew in the family." I imagined the canopy, and I knew I had been fooling myself. Danny was taking a vacation from his life: dating me, eating shellfish, watching cartoons. He wasn't going to give up his faith for lobster. I saw my revised plate for the years to come: baked potato, corn, a roll. And Danny. Was it enough? In the end, it didn't matter. The relationship sputtered, faded into something else. I got to keep my friend Danny, and I got to keep my lobster. Sometimes I still wonder what my decision would have been.

⁘

LOBSTERS FADED INTO the background of my life for a few years, barely causing a ripple of memory when I saw them on menus. Life in the corporate world took its toll on my joy and my health, and I, like my father so many years before, realized that I needed an escape. I left my job and enrolled in cooking school, taking the first step on a path that would lead me back to lobsters.

Day Ten of cooking school. Already I have dumped a quart of chicken stock into my partner's knife kit, slashed my finger open and bled all over a case of onions. But I, who have been known to get weepy because of a rude mail carrier or a maudlin long-distance commercial, am determined not to cry. My chef-instructor asks the class, "Has anyone cooked lobsters before?" I raise my hand. Finally, something I can do.

Boiling lobsters never threw me. I'd watched my parents do it so often that I didn't flinch the first time I threw my own Chinatown-bought lobsters into a boiling pot in my kitchen on Avenue A. It wasn't exactly the Maine coast, but they still tasted good. Lobsters were my first indication that, for me to eat, something had to die. Though I was a painfully sensitive child, the cold facts of carnivorism didn't bother little Gretchen in the slightest. The lobsters went in the pot kicking and came out delicious, and that was the way of the world.

"Okay, so you know that the tail and the claws should be cooked separately, right?" the chef asked.

"Um, okay . . ."

"So you'll need to take apart these ten lobsters for me."

"Take . . . apart?"

"So you've never done this," he said, staring at me.

"I guess not."

He grabbed two towels, held the front section of a lobster in his left hand, the back section in his right, and twisted, hard. In a second, there were two squirming lobster halves on the table. "Got it?" he asked me.

"Got it," I said through clenched teeth. I had boiled dozens of lobsters without a thought, but somehow dismemberment was another story. *They're bugs,* I told myself. *Big, ugly bugs. You can step on a cockroach, right? So you can kill a lobster.*

I wound the towels around my hands and approached the smallest, most sluggish lobster on the pile. I flinched, let a tear drop down my cheek. The chef saw it, but said nothing. I picked up the lobster, twisted. "Harder. Do it fast. Twist. Now!" I did it. Made two pieces of lobster out of a live lobster. "Good. Now do the next one." The second one was hard. The fifth was almost easy. And the tenth was like chopping a carrot. Freedom from compassion in ten easy lessons, thanks to a hard-ass chef.

Four months later, I found myself working the *garde-manger* station at a lively East Village bistro. The lobster salad was a very popular summer item, and within a few weeks I could turn a dozen cooked lobsters into salad meat in ten minutes flat. Dragging my tired body home on the subway late one night, I realized that the crowds of riders were giving me a wide berth. That

exotic undersea perfume in the air—that was me. I was morti-
fied. And a little bit proud.

Saltwater runs through my blood, after all. That first taste of
lobster had contributed more to my fate and my choices than anyone might have guessed. I am the daughter of a lobsterman/paper
executive and a first-grade teacher who can cook a mean loaf of
SPAM. My plate runneth over with sweet corn; a brown Russet
potato slashed open to reveal floury, buttered insides; a crisp sourdough roll; and a bright red Long Island Sound lobster, claws dangling over the side, just waiting for me to dig in.

gripes of wrath

{ SUZANNE HAMLIN }

I KNOW I LOOK old enough to order wine. So why, when I go out to dinner with friends, am I almost never offered a wine list? For that matter, why is it that there is only one list for the entire table? After all, everybody gets a menu, glasses, silverware, napkins. Why should just one person be empowered to order the wine that everyone will be drinking—and perhaps paying for, too?

Here we are at The French Laundry, in Napa, for example, all of us eagerly anticipating our annual reunion with Thomas Keller's food. The staff knows us (it's hard to forget a sextet of diners who appear once a year to eat at least twenty-three courses over the course of six hours), and we know and adore them. But when the sommelier appears with the beautifully seductive wine list, he goes directly to one person. Okay, the chosen one is a wine writer whose talent is unquestioned, but some of the best food and wine writers I know are also sitting—now literally listless—at the same table.

While the sommelier and the list-holder engage in a lengthy dialogue, including personal reminiscences about a particular Alsace winemaker, the rest of us turn to each other and wait it out. Finally, several wines are anointed and we begin the meal. Enjoyment is not a question here, but by around course fifteen none of us knows exactly what we're drinking; the delicious wines, whose names we have never seen written out, have become a blur. Yes, they are red and they are white. But are they from Sonoma or Croatia? Are they small, exclusive bottlings or widely available? The only detail we sharers of the bill ultimately remember is the price.

I've asked restaurateurs and wine professionals just why this old-fashioned French restaurant scenario still takes place in an age of relative enlightenment in the areas of wine and service. Some of the answers have been sensible, some have been bogus, and some have been downright hostile.

At just about any restaurant fancier than a diner, the one-list-per-table rule is in effect; who is picked to actually receive the list has little more logic than the lottery. As two sommeliers explained to me, the list is given to the person who answers "Yes" first to the question, "Will you be having wine tonight?" If everyone nods yes, the waiter uses "body language" to determine who the wine contact at the table will be. Confronted with a hard-to-read or passive table, the waiter usually resorts to the drop-and-run technique, putting the list down on a neutral part of the table and letting the best grabber win.

The victor—your friend, lover, client, boss—essentially becomes your wine director for the evening. In short, you have been relegated to the equivalent of the children's table, along with the other enologically challenged dimwits you're dining with.

"Amazing, isn't it? The sommelier still decides who the adult at the table is," says Joyce Goldstein, cutting to the chase when I call her for comment. Goldstein, the outspoken and innovative San Francisco restaurateur, author, and consultant, simply did for others what she wanted for herself during the twelve-year life span of her restaurant, Square One. Everybody got a copy of the wine list, updated two or three times a week. (During a California paper-saving campaign in the mid-'90s, it was cut back to one list for every two diners.)

This freedom-of-wine-information fight, in addition to increasing fun and pleasure, also helps eliminate the lingering sexism that taints wine service. Mary Ewing-Mulligan, president of the International Wine Center, in New York, relates with a kind of bemused resignation her dining experiences with her husband, Ed McCarthy, a wine writer. "If the restaurant knows us, we're each given a list; if they don't, invariably it's handed to Ed."

⋯⋰⋯

THE UNILATERAL SOLUTION seems so simple: one diner, one menu, one wine list, no problems.

But maybe you don't really care about the wine list. Maybe you know nothing about wine, or think you know nothing, or consider choosing it intimidating. But if you drink wine, you should care, even if someone else will finally decide what the table is drinking. A wine list tells you a lot about a restaurant, about its own adventurous spirit (or lack of one), about its price structure, its respect for its patrons, or—I'm looking right now at one such banal, overpriced list—its cynicism. Most of all, a good list will introduce you to grapes and wines you've never heard of. Assuming that the staff is at least somewhat knowledgeable, consider it a free learning opportunity.

Increasingly, trattorias and bistros combine the menu and the wine list; a good look that, not surprisingly, usually boosts wine sales. But is an inordinately large list a legitimate excuse for a restaurant to do the wrong thing? Anyone who has ever seen the wine list at Sparks Steak House, a meat mecca in Manhattan with a breathtakingly deep list of reds, knows that size doesn't really matter. The Sparks menu and wine list are one, a printed miracle of sorts that sets an industry standard.

Really, though, how difficult would it be for most restaurants to simply hand one menu and one wine list to each diner? If you're not interested, don't bother to look at it. Maybe someday you'll get tired of not looking at it. Mary Ewing-Mulligan is convinced that if someone hands you something over and over again, you're eventually going to read it. Maybe you'll learn something, and maybe you'll lose the feeling that wine is a subject open only to a few. Maybe it will lead to a spirited discussion around the table about wine.

And that, of course, is what it's all about. Or should be.

not up to haute cuisine

{ CHRISTINA HENRY DE TESSAN }

ONE EVENING, ON a recent trip to Paris, I found myself alone and looking for a place to dine. Free to select a restaurant on my own—without any companions to hint that I should be making the most of being in France by eating at some classic brasserie—I made my way to the bustling, aromatic Italian trattoria down the street from where I was staying. A jovial Italian waiter ushered me in, pulled a table out for me, presented me with the menu, and rushed off to pour me a glass of the house red. As I sat, choosing between a delicate truffle-infused risotto and a fiery pasta Puttanesca, I considered the fact that once again, I found myself in a non-French restaurant in one of the great food capitals of the world—this restaurant choice was quite clearly part of a greater pattern. Whenever I was in Paris, I routinely managed to slip past the French restaurants with their unorthodox cuts of meat blanketed by bland cream sauces in my quest for more exotic, flavorful fare. At Pirosmani, a tiny Georgian restaurant, the beef stew hinted at nuts and cinnamon, which I devoured with steaming *khachapuri,* a kind of cheese turnover, and full-bodied Georgian red wine. My favorite stop at the outdoor market was the Lebanese merchant, who made thin-crusted breads brushed with lemon and thyme over a heated convex metal drum right before my eyes. Time and again, I found myself seeking out "foreign" food—in the very birthplace of haute cuisine.

The fact is that I don't think much of classic Parisian food. This in itself would not matter much except that I am French—or, more correctly, my father is French, born in Paris, and he cares deeply about his country's great culinary tradition. Whether he is simmering tender little *rognons* (veal kidneys) in cream or slathering a great swab of *rillettes* (shredded pork meat and fat) on bread, each meal is an opportunity to honor that tradition. Fiercely loyal to his small, unwavering stock of top-quality ingredients and a narrow repertoire of recipes, he cares nothing for the various food trends that come and go, instead focusing on perfecting dishes he already knows well. All my life, he has plucked the choicest morsels from various bits of offal and held them before my eyes, begging for a glimmer of enthusiasm. When I am invited over for dinner and asked with gusto whether I would enjoy some fine *foie de veau* (calf's liver), I weakly decline, wishing that I could match his passion for the cuisine of his childhood. He sighs, baffled at my lack of appreciation. When it came time to size up my fiancé, my father dared him to join him in ordering calf's head off the menu at a traditional French bistro. The iron-stomached fiancé heartily agreed, and the final seal of approval was granted.

In an era that's all about finding our roots and bringing back traditional cooking methods, and as someone who has a great deal of reverence for food, I have always been something of a disappointment to myself, if not my father. How proud he would be if

I would tuck into a bit of tripe, expound on the magnificent texture of a blood sausage, or express suitable awe at a perfect *sauce béarnaise*. How I would love to be less squeamish about the meats, and more awed by the flavors, of such a noble culinary heritage. But again and again, I find myself gravitating toward other, infinitely sexier cuisines and flavors. Given the choice, I would happily select fish tacos sprinkled with onion, cilantro, and a splash of lime over a formally plated steak and *pommes de terre sautés*.

❖

As I sat in my lovely trattoria savoring the bitter and salty pairing of baked radicchio wrapped in pancetta, I wondered whether this preference for foods other than French has less to do with flavor than with context, and whether my childhood memories have truly shaped my palate. My father moved to San Francisco in his late twenties, where he has lived ever since, but his family remains in Paris. As a child, I went once a year to visit my grandmother and other relatives, a volatile lot who managed never to get along but always to gather for a command performance when Dad came to town, creating further opportunities for discord.

During these visits, I was made to sit through endless, formal meals with my extended family: my fiercely anti-elitest aunt dressed in plain home-sewn cotton dresses; her pedantically Catholic husband; my Americanized father and American mother; my kind but somewhat deaf great-aunt who spoke in strident tones; her gentle, formal husband; and, of course, my grandmother. In the silk-lined dining room, where weighty silver candelabras rose grandly out of the center of the long rectangular table, my formidable grandmother, draped in great ropes of gold necklaces and sparkling with gems, held court at the head of the table. While my grandmother desperately tried to preserve the formalities of the old regime, her children wanted nothing more than to escape its confines. All she'd ever wanted was to have her children marry those of her friends, live in one of two appropriate neighborhoods a few minutes away, and invite her to Sunday lunch for the rest of her life. As it turned out, her daughter fled to the countryside and her two sons moved across the Atlantic and married foreigners. But rather than enjoying these dinners with her children, our reunions supplied her with a rare opportunity to steep them in guilt for having abandoned her. A refrain of *"je suis seule au monde"* (I am alone in the world) punctuated every conversation.

Meanwhile, the *gigot d'agneau* (leg of lamb) and *pommes de terre sautés* (potatoes), pasty *flageolets*, and an array of cheeses, were passed on sparkling silver platters by patient help and subjected to the most meticulous criticism: "The lamb is tough—and not pink enough." Or, it was the cheese that came under fire: "The Camembert isn't sufficiently ripe." Sometimes it was *too* ripe and simply declared *"inmangeable"* (inedible). Then it was time for dessert: *"Sans goût. Absolument sans aucun goût."* (Flavorless. Absolutely flavorless.) Then Grand-mère would declare that she hated dessert anyway, and ask for some yogurt to be brought. (I, on the other hand, always found dessert delightful. Sometimes it took the form of a strawberry tart, with the glazed red fruit set in perfect, ever-widening circles. Occasionally, there was ice cream, which was sliced into perfect rectangles on the plate rather than scooped casually into bowls.) In part, my grandmother's dissection of the meal took place because she, like so many Parisians of her generation, swapped her loyalty for preferential treatment from the merchants she frequented, and in her world, a poor cut of meat was an insult. In any case, there was little joy to be wrung from this food, as perfection proved ever elusive.

In this staid setting, neatly dressed in my plaid kilt and itchy tights, often half-delirious from jet lag, I swung my legs back and forth, pushed the food around my plate with my oversized silverware, and waited quietly for dessert. I was too young to understand the subtle, but stinging, remarks that were volleyed back and forth across the table, but I could sense the tension in the voices of the adults. The heightened formality at the table was not designed to put anyone at ease, but instead to impress and intimidate. And intimidate it certainly did. This was not a room that invited exuberant chatter and raucous laughter, and not a group prone to either. Childish giggles were out of the question. Even at the best of times, when everyone was determined to behave, dinner tended to be a long and solemn affair—it was a group graced with little humor and who lacked that French quality of joie de vivre. As I was too young to partake of either the wine or the family arguments, these made for long evenings. It's clear that the memory of those evenings still lingers on my palate.

⁛

FORTUNATELY, WHEN I was not in Paris being subjected to the rigid formalities of Parisian high society, I lived in San Francisco, which was a food-obsessed town even then, so I was lucky enough to be exposed to a chaotic abundance of flavors from across the globe. Food was in, limitless ingredients were at hand, and my mother was an avid—and highly successful—adventurer in the kitchen. From a young age, I savored shrimp stir-fries exploding with ginger and scallions, fluffy and buttery couscous, steaming risottos dotted with mushrooms and sprinkled with fresh Parmesan. I slurped up Asian noodles slippery with sesame oil in my school lunch, burned my tongue on steamed pork buns outside the Ashby BART station after school, tasted the smoky flavor of Hungarian paprika sprinkled over chicken when I spent the night in the Berkeley Hills at my best friend's house, and casually feasted on curries and warm Indian naan at slumber parties.

My American grandmother lived on Russian Hill in a small apartment with soaring views over the Bay, and was an excellent, if haphazard, cook, whose fingers were scarred with countless cuts from her kitchen knives and who liked to joke that the wine would breathe faster if she ran it through the Cuisinart. For family dinners, we outfitted the card table in her small dining room with a large round table top that she kept hidden under her bed, and pulled out folding chairs from the pantry. It was a cozy arrangement— once seated, you couldn't get up without disrupting everyone else. From a kitchen the size of a closet—where cooking equipment was stacked in teetering columns to the ceiling and in the oven— emerged the most glorious dishes. She was especially famous for her Chinese chicken salad, my favorite part of it being the miraculous translucent noodles that puffed up like Styrofoam when dropped in hot oil. My cousin Patrick and I were often in charge of dessert, which consisted of walking down to Swensens at Hyde and Union and ordering Sticky Chewy Chocolate ice cream by the quart. On Chili Sundays, everyone heaped their bowls with spicy steaming chili, sprinkled with sour cream, cilantro, and cheese, and found a spot on the bed or floor in front of the TV in my grandmother's bedroom to watch her beloved 49ers win or lose.

When my uncle came into town with my many cousins, we always reserved two large round tables at Mike's Chinese Cuisine, where we traumatized the other clientele with raucous conversation and cascades of laughter. The lazy susan spun round and round, a dizzying array of Mongolian beef, mushrooms in oyster sauce, Peking duck, fried rice, pot stickers, spring rolls, and sizzling shrimp all vanishing within minutes. It was at one of these boisterous free-for-alls that I learned to use chopsticks for the first time—a good thing because although I never went hungry, you couldn't be shy at these family affairs, and it helped to be quick.

It was always dizzying, chaotic—and I remember those days fondly. I was younger than most of the group at the table, and sat with rapt awe as the group jostled and laughed and drank and ate its way through those meals. It was impossible to keep up, but I soaked up the jovial atmosphere and the festive spirit that my glamorous New York relatives inspired in everyone around them. To this day, I order Chinese chicken salad and Mongolian beef whenever they are on the menu, ever hopeful that I will be able to replicate the experience of feasting on them in such joyful company.

❖

AFTER FINISHING MY thimbleful of espresso at my Italian trattoria, I paid the check. As I walked back to my hotel through the narrow streets, I remembered a silly promise I'd made to myself on my thirtieth birthday: I would stop pretending to like things only because I was supposed to. And the time had arrived to come clean: The French could continue to lord their culinary heritage over the world, but I didn't have to like it—despite the French blood that courses through my veins. They could take their centuries of meticulous techniques and traditions: their finely puréed sauces; their endless ways of preparing potatoes; their fear of spices; their languid, overcooked vegetables; their unappealing cuts of meat and complicated methods of preparing them; and they could enjoy them all with gusto—and without me. Thankfully, my father has taken this all in stride, especially now that he has found a kindred spirit in my husband, who is willing to tuck into a calf's head and praise the merits of tripe when called upon to do so.

When my American grandmother died a few years ago, I inherited her cooking utensils and cookbooks. This seems like a symbolic gift as well as a practical one, since it's the unlikely American side of my family, with its chaotic, eclectic, adventurous way with food that ultimately won my culinary allegiance. Better to experiment with joy than strive for perfection without. Of course, the French probably wouldn't agree.

being food

{ M A R I A N N E   A P O S T O L I D E S }

THE WOMAN WAS *pregnant, and wasting away. In her ethereal weakness, she climbed a kitchen chair each morning to look into her neighbor's garden. There among the beans and beets grew wet, emerald rampion— a lettuce-like vegetable common to Germany. She pined for the rampion, but knew she could never taste it, for her neighbor was a witch both quiet and fierce.*

Because the woman so desired the rampion, she would eat nothing else, and fell into the swirling delirium of slow starvation.

After several helpless weeks, the woman's husband risked his life to creep into the witch's garden and steel an armful of the ripe roughage.

When he returned home, his wife held the rampion against her cheek. Its leaves were soft, like a new baby's skin. That very night, in her kitchen lit by the moon, the woman ate a salad as large as a cooking pot. But when the rampion ran out, she grew hungry once more. And so her husband returned to the witch's garden.

He had gathered almost a dozen plants when he heard a low, steady laughter behind him. The witch was sitting on a bench, watching him with eyes that glistened as green as the rampion.

"Don't worry," she said in a voice creaky from disuse. "You may have all the rampion your wife desires."

"Thank you," the man whispered as he backed up and began to run confusedly, changing direction like a frightened rabbit.

"But," the witch called after him, trapping him with her voice, "you must first promise to give me your child . . . if she is a girl."

Without turning to face the witch, the man agreed, knowing he would have neither child nor wife if he did not nourish his wife with the rampion.

For the next six months the woman thrived. Finally the baby was born—a perfect child, a girl child. That very night, the witch strolled into the house and took the child off her mother's breast. "I will name you after the food that brought you to me," she cooed as she walked away, ignoring the cries of the parents. And so the girl was known by the German word for rampion; and so the girl was known as Rapunzel.

⁙

ONLY LATER IN the story, when the girl had grown up beautifully on the food from the witch's garden, did Rapunzel let down her golden hair.

Rapunzel is one of the many folk tales recorded by Jakob and Wilhelm Grimm, those early folklorists who traveled through Germany capturing the oral tales of their culture. "Who but a pregnant woman would crave like that?" the German people seemed to say in this tale—a story retold by generations of women as they worked together to wash potatoes, chop carrots, and stir stews that slowly submitted to the heat of red flames.

⁙

UNLIKE RAPUNZEL'S FABLED mother, I didn't want roughage at the beginning of my pregnancy. At first, I craved orange juice. I wanted it to wet my mouth, to keep its sun beside my tongue and cheeks. For weeks, I drank gallons of it, eventually squeezing my own from dozens of orange globes. The liquid would rush from its thick encasement, pooling in a well from which I drank directly, foregoing a glass. A soft breath of citrus would perfume my fingers all day, teasing me as I adjusted my glasses or brushed back the hair from my face.

With that initial craving, I was being led, belly first, into that unique state known as pregnancy. I was now food.

No one can explain definitively why women feel cravings during pregnancy, or why most experience morning sickness. Researchers have postulated that the hormone hCG, produced by the developing placenta, causes nausea. But this theory has never been proven; the mystery remains wrapped inside women's bodies.

In the medical literature, morning sickness has not been linked directly with cravings. But as I slid an unexpectedly smooth course between nausea and desire, I knew with simple clarity that these two phenomena were interlocked. Without that awful, burbling nausea, I could not have felt those specific, insistent cravings, or the elation that came with fulfilling them. To me, it is clear that the unknown underlying cause of both is the same. "Morning sickness" would be more properly described as a full-on bodily experience of food—the good and the bad.

I believe this experience arises, at least indirectly, from the augmentation of our sense of taste. When I became pregnant, I felt as if I had entered a whole other sensory realm—a dimension of the world that exists parallel to ours, unknown to all but pregnant women. I could describe this realm with synesthetic language: flavors were bright, or cascading, or trumpeting. But I can best give *evidence* of this realm by describing the abrupt change in the sense most linked to taste: the sense of smell.

When I was pregnant, I could smell far beyond my usual capacity. I didn't quite appreciate the extent of the augmentation until a walk at dusk on a hot July night. My husband and I were strolling through the neighborhood when our little dog spun and squatted and pooed. "My god!" I said. "That one stinks!"

My husband said nothing as he walked across the lawn toward our dog. I remained on the sidewalk fifteen feet away, my nose crinkled in displeasure, while my husband bent to scoop the offending waste. "I didn't smell it till now," he said.

We resumed our walk. As I watched the dog's nose follow the urban tracks of squirrels and French fries, I realized I was temporarily closer to my canine than my husband in terms of smell. Our dog roamed through the same space we did, but knew an entirely different world—a world of black-and-white visions, with a brilliant spectrum of smells. I was now privy to that universe.

By the same underlying mystery, I was also privy to a new universe of desire and taste. Before I became pregnant, I had some vague, kooky notion of the reality of women's cravings: peanut butter on pasta at 5:00 A.M. *That* would be a craving.

But the experience wasn't crazy at all. Cravings were simply an intensification of a process we feel all the time: an unconscious checking-in with the body's desires for tastes and nutrients. We go through this process when deciding whether to have split-pea soup or *aloo gobi*; whether to have chamomile or Darjeeling tea. But this process of deciding what to eat can often take place in our heads—what we *think* we should eat. And even when we try to check in with our bodies, the signals can often be too faint to read.

Pregnancy eliminated any ambiguity in food preferences. My body's signals become booming, operatic announcements of culinary desire and repulsion. By smelling random ingredients, I could determine exactly what my body needed. I knew when I wanted blackberry jam with crunchy peanut butter on multigrain bread: not blueberry jam, but blackberry; not smooth peanut butter, but crunchy; not whole wheat bread, but multigrain—the one with flax seeds, not caraway. The very fact of knowing was a freedom, and thrilled my body like the first breeze of spring. I did not care what the preference was—whether chocolate cake or black beans, sweet or savory—I cared only that I knew my preference with such easy certainty.

When I listened to my body's messages, even the crudest meals became a complexity of sensations percolating through my receptive taste buds. Food tasted different; it tasted somehow . . . bigger. For me, the difference between eating and eating during early pregnancy was like the difference between having sex and having sex with an orgasm. It was a new level of eating, deeper and higher at the same time, not sexual but fully body, every muscle engaged for me, asking nothing in response.

This fleeting moment of orgasmic eating reached its climax when I was halfway through my first trimester, not yet showing but firmly feeling myself as a pregnant woman. I sat cross-legged on the bed with my husband, eating baked potatoes with melted cheese and a kiss of salt and pepper. We now delighted in the dawning understanding that we would soon become parents, that we had already linked our bodies in the unceasing embrace that is a child.

We talked lightly about our hopes as we ate the white earth of the round potatoes. "I'm not full," I said, looking at my empty plate.

"What would you like?" he asked. At that moment, I couldn't pinpoint the food, just its tastes—sweet but salty, warm and crunchy, but *real* food, not a snack. I couldn't quite grasp what that food was, but my husband could. Without a word, he disappeared to create something that would nourish me and our baby. I lay back in bed, listening to the kitchen beat in time to the knife's controlled dance.

Soon my *channa*-making, bread-baking, gourmet-cooking

husband arrived back in the bedroom. Upon the plate lay a modest, flat sandwich.

"Grilled cheese," he declared.

Ornery old cheddar cheese melted under languid onions and splayed tomatoes, all held between the firm hands of crisp bread toasted over the skillet's black heat.

This grilled cheese sandwich was the pinnacle of my gustatory life, thanks somehow to my little girl who was still too little to be a girl; to my body perfect in its knowing; to my husband for both listening and cooking; and to me for eating each bite in the unconscious bliss of true awareness.

⚜

THE CRAVINGS AND nausea dissipated as my pregnancy progressed. The absence of those insistent phenomena created a calm space where I could finally touch the epiphany that forever changed my relationship to food.

From far back in childhood, I had heard "you are what you eat" and "food is your fuel." But those words strung together had become hollow sounds, holding no meaning.

Now, any abstraction surrounding food was eliminated: I took food into my mouth, silently broke it down into its nutrients, then incorporated those unseen components visibly into my body, into my baby who grew over my core. My outstretched belly—a lush roundness from which I could hear my baby's heartbeat and feel her undulations—was a physical manifestation of food becoming me. The connection between me and food was finally clear: Food is my flesh and my spirit, my blood and my pulse. Food is inseparable from self.

And so it was during my pregnancy that I finally chose to become a vegetarian who eats organic food. Four years later, I still eat only vegetables and fruits grown without chemical spray, in soil containing no human sludge, unmodified by science. These foods grew on their own time, taking what they needed from the fertile soil around them. These foods grew just like the child inside me.

After each visit to our midwife, my husband and I shopped at the local organic foods store. We walked among the many-colored jewels of the earth—slender beans that reached toward fennel with its wispy hair; aggressive jalapeños that gathered beside eggplants, plump and stately in their purple skin. The store was a paradise separate from the grit of the city. Here, food was respected; here, I felt the connection between the distant soil worked by farmers and the food I ate at my table each night. As I placed different vegetables in a bin, recipes wrote themselves in my mind. I would now learn to combine these foods, to coax them into releasing their subtle tastes in my mouth.

·❖·

MY BABY GOT bigger, and so did I. I wore my clothes tight over my gorgeous belly, my body announcing that I was nurturing a life. I felt the freedom of this bursting body, ripening everywhere. That body was not mine to consider "fat" or "thin." That body was hers—her home in which to find the space and rhythm and warmth in order to become.

During pregnancy, my baby was fed by my blood. By the time I was at term, the volume of my blood had increased by 50 percent, and my heart muscle was pumping one-third harder to send that redness through the rivers of my body and into my child. My veins and arteries entered the placenta, offering blood to be absorbed by fetal capillaries that ran toward my baby's umbilical cord. Through this tough white tunnel, blood rushed into the fetus's core, giving her nutrients, water, and oxygen—giving her all she needed to grow from a wish into an eight-pound baby with her own perfect body and mind.

⁙

SHE WAS BORN under a full moon on the first day of spring. Now I would feed her from without, from my milk instead of my blood. I have become used to the idea that my breasts produce milk, but when I first saw my own milk leaving my body, I felt I was witness to the sacred.

In those first few weeks of my child's life, her only sense of calm and satisfaction came from my body. My breastmilk nourished her for months, responding to her needs, producing more or less according to the natural curve of her growth. She knew when to eat, and asked for food with her cries or her body's reach toward my breast; she knew, too, when to stop, releasing her latch to look at my face, or falling into serene sleep.

Similarly, my body knew what to make—what mixture of fat and sugar, which vitamins and in what concentration. A woman's foremilk is always sweet, higher in simple sugars to give her baby a hit of energy, to keep the child awake and sucking long enough to get the hindmilk—the creamier milk higher in fat and protein, the milk that makes babies grow at such exponential rates. Throughout a child's infancy, the composition of hindmilk changes, carrying different nutrients in different proportions according to the developmental needs of the child.

The milk was made inside my breasts, in clusters of cells which turned nutrients from my blood into a thin, pearly stream. When my baby suckled, her lips and gums compressed my nipple, sending signals that told my breast to make and release milk. My child then took this sweetness, drawing it into her mouth with her strong tongue. Through this connection between her body and mine— a connection most animal and most godly—my milk nourished my baby. Every strengthened muscle and lengthened bone, all new knowledge of senses and self, came first from the food that my body provided.

In this age of formula and breast-pumping, I could have been apart from my child during those first six months. But I chose not to be. For a half year, she ate only of me, and only from my breasts. She emerged as her own self—the violated, vulnerable newborn settling into a curious being capable of delight and humor, disappointment and joy. But until I gave her that first bite of cereal, she was still me.

grilled cheese sandwich

Bread

Butter

Cheese (any kind you like; I prefer a sharp cheddar)

Onion

Tomato

Slice four pieces of bread. Lay them on the counter. Butter the top sides of the bread. Take every other slice of bread and flip it onto the slice next to it. (You will therefore have buttered side atop buttered side). Slice the cheese as thick or thin as you like. Cover the (unbuttered) top sides of the bread with the cheese. Cut rounds of the onion as thin as you can. Place them on the cheese. Cut rounds of tomato as thin as you can. Place them on the onion. Pick up the two assembled top pieces. Put them (bread-side down) in a medium-hot skillet or frying pan. Put the other slices of bread on top of the assembled pieces, so the buttered side is up. Press down on the sandwich with a spatula, squishing the fully assembled sandwich. When the bottom bread is golden with caramel-brown veins and speckles, flip the sandwiches over. (As you flip, you may need to hold the sandwich together with your fingers.) Squish again. Check for browning. Eat 'em while they're hot.

carvel

{ E L I Z A B E T H N U N E Z }

Ï AM AN unremorseful ice cream addict, still unremorseful even after the day I almost traded my life for an ice-cream
cone. It was not an ordinary ice-cream cone, to be sure, that almost
cost me my life, though you, dear reader, would probably call it
ordinary. But to me it was, *is*, the Picasso of ice creams, the Aretha
Franklin of ice creams, the James Baldwin of ice creams, the
Beethoven of ice creams, the Edna Lewis of ice creams, the pinnacle, the apotheosis of ice creams. A Carvel soft-serve ice cream
on a pale, biscuit-color wafer cone: the kind of ice cream that curls
out of a metal spigot from the upright, plastic machine in the Carvel
ice-cream parlor, the kind of wafer cone that disintegrates in your
hand if held too indelicately, if approached with too much anxiety.

Yes, I am familiar with designer ice creams. I have a reputation
for having a somewhat sophisticated palate. I set a good table and
flatter myself with being someone who, though not in the league

of Julia Child, could be regarded as a disciple. But when it comes to ice cream, only Carvel will do. I love its simplicity. In a world that can bring us to the brink of psychic distress with the dizzying array of daily choices we must make—even something as mundane as toilet paper comes in a rainbow of colors, textures and scents—Carvel is wonderfully reassuring. They offer only two ice-cream flavors at Carvel, vanilla or chocolate, though for the more intrepid, and sometimes I have been intrepid, there is the swirl, chocolate and vanilla rising in a glorious dance up a mountain. And what a mountain! Marge Simpson's hair balancing precariously on her head, a tiny cowlick finishing it off at the peak. And what a cone! Crumbling in defiance of the plastic mold intended to hold its shape the minute teeth sink into it, so that the wafer breaks to bits in your hand and ice cream snakes unceremoniously down your fingers.

I know all the Carvel ice-cream parlors within a five-mile radius of my home. I know when they open and, more importantly, when they close, so that in the middle of the night, should I hear the call of the ice-cream siren, I know where to go. I have no sailors to lash me to a ship's mast, as they did poor Odysseus. I can be safely ensconced in my bed, in my nightgown, my down comforter drawn snugly up to my chin, but I will still answer her, so seductive is she to me, so strong is my addiction. I have known winters when the snow was piled high at my doorway and the weatherman was warning of blustery winds and temperatures below zero, and yet the ice-cream siren has lured me. I pull on sweater and sweat pants over my nightgown, I jump in my car, I make my way across slippery roads, caring not a whit for my safety.

At the college where I teach, I once foolishly confessed my addiction to the cashier in the cafeteria. She is a fat woman, perennially on a diet, and I am fairly slim. I eat what I want for lunch and she envies me this indulgence. But on Wednesdays, I eat only fat-free pretzels; I drink only tea without sugar. The cashier seems secretly pleased when I present these to her at the register. She gives me her widest smile. One day, she said to me conspiratorially, "I see you are on one, too."

"One?" I asked.

"Diet," she said and practically winked at me.

"Oh, no. Wednesday is sundae at Carvel," I answered. She looked at me, puzzled. "Sunday?" she asked. I spelled it out for her. She has since stopped smiling at me.

I have no dinner on Wednesdays, either. It is a diet of sorts, I guess, that I inflict on myself in exchange for the joys to come later that evening. "No, it's not necessary to put a cover on it," I say to the young woman who serves me the ice-cream sundae. She shrugs, figures I am some sort of oddball, a kook, and asks, "Sprinkles? Nuts? Syrup?"

A sane person would want sprinkles, nuts or syrup, she seems to imply with raised eyebrows. Not me. I know how I like my Carvel's. I want it pure, untainted.

"Sure you want the other one the same way?" she asks. On Wednesdays, you get two sundaes for the price of one.

After my purchase, I race home, put one in the freezer, drop my handbag and briefcase on the floor, take off my coat and shoes, stretch out on my sofa and pig out, my pleasure quadrupled by the sure knowledge that there is another Carvel sundae waiting for me in the freezer after I get into my night clothes.

Where and when did this all begin, this addiction I have neither the intention nor the motivation to curb? How did ice cream, Carvel ice cream, become so irresistible to me that a day would come when I would offer my head on a platter, willingly, just for that exquisite sensation, so irresistible to me, when my tongue, hot and moist, glides over the sweet, creamy coolness of a spiraling tower of soft serve and balances on its tip a small, gooey mound that I guide slowly down the warmth of my throat?

I have only to shut my eyes and it comes back to me: those Sunday afternoons in the sweltering heat of the tropical sun in Trinidad, the place of my birth. My mother is making ice cream, as she does every Sunday after lunch. Early in the morning, one of my brothers would have cut open a dried coconut and scooped out the hardened flesh. My older sister would have grated it, put it into a basin with just enough boiling water to release the coconut juices, and then strained it. Now, my mother mixes the coconut juice with condensed milk, evaporated milk, and custard powder (three tins each of the milk and two tablespoons of the custard). On the stove, a pot of water (three cups) is boiling. My mother has already made a paste with cornstarch (two tablespoons) and a little water, and she deftly whisks it into the boiling water. When the water thickens with the cornstarch, she adds the milk, coconut juice, and custard mixture, lets it all thicken some more, and then takes the pot off the stove. The last ingredient is gelatin. "Just enough," my mother says, "to give the ice cream a smooth taste." I know that taste, silk coursing down the canal of my throat, soothing my tonsils that are constantly inflamed, I am certain by the heat.

The churning is next. Before the churning, directly after lunch, my father would have gone with my brothers to the ice-cream factory and they will have brought back a block of ice which they have covered with a crocus bag. Now that the ice-cream mixture is ready, my mother pours it in the container inside the ice-cream maker. My brothers chip away the block of ice with an ice pick and pack the pieces around the container, a layer of ice followed by a layer of salt.

I am too young to churn the ice-cream maker, but at six or seven I am old enough to "fend" (to defend my claim) for the ladle inside the container. This day I "outfend" my older sister and brother and once the ice-cream has hardened, my mother pulls out the ladle and hands it to me. I sit in the shade of the mango tree in our back yard, and I lick it dry. Soon the skin around my mouth is matted with the sweet stickiness of coconut ice cream; little trails of white run down my chin, past my neck into the top of my dress. At times in my search for the creamy sweetness that lies lodged in the grill of the ladle, my tongue encounters cold metal. Sometimes it sticks. It is part of the pleasure: the cold, the sweetness, the hot sun, the sting of the metal, the joy of my mother's homemade coconut ice-cream filling every cavity of my body. If there is a heaven, I think, this must be what it promises.

-:::-

ON THAT FRIGHTENING afternoon, as I drove to my breast surgeon to get the results of my mammogram, six months after a surgical bioscopy revealed I had an in situ malignancy (zero stage cancer, my breast surgeon called it, but to me, *cancer*), I longed for those carefree days, those ice-cream days, when I was safe, when I was happy and secure, when my breasts threatened me with no more than the stubborn flatness of two round brown spots that I feared would never grow into the luscious loaves rising on my mother's chest.

The traffic was thick. I was in a busy intersection in Queens, New York, the third car back stopped at the traffic light. To both my right and left traffic whizzed past me nonstop. I saw this vaguely, for my mind was clouded with fear of what I was certain my breast surgeon would say to me: "I am sorry, Elizabeth." (My mother is in remission for breast cancer; her mother died of it.) As panic choked me, I grasped for a straw, for a memory. Ice cream. I turned my head to the left. Even to this day, I do not know why. I know only that I felt an irresistible urge to turn my head to the left, and there it was: Carvel, my Carvel, rising heroically before me. I twisted my wheel and stepped on the gas.

The man who hit me was confounded by my reaction: I had gotten out of the car and walked like a zombie into the ice-cream parlor, seemingly heedless of the curses he was hurling upon me. "A soft-serve swirl in a wafer cone," I said to the astonished fresh-faced girl. "Large." The man screamed at me. His words rolled past my ears like water off a duck's back.

The manager of the store came out from the back room. He had heard the commotion. "A large soft-serve swirl in a wafer cone," I repeated. He stared at me in amazement. The man who hit me yelled louder now. He was a countryman, Trinidadian born, like me. His face was contorted with anger and frustration. "She *crazy!* She must be crazy. I nearly kill she and she saying, 'Large. I want a large one.'"

Only when I felt the ice cream fill my mouth with its cold sweetness did clarity return.

⁘

MY BREAST SURGEON said I looked like a woman who had taken some happy-making drug. She didn't trust the smile on my face. She took me by the hand and put me to sit in her office. I looked scary, she said, but happy.

my mother's kitchen

{ AMANDA SULLIVAN }

IT IS CHRISTMAS Eve and I am cooking in my mother's kitchen. Before the holiday is done I will have "walked a mile" in her shoes, as the saying goes.

If I don't pull out the china and shine the silver at least once a year, I worry that some part of my mother will mysteriously disappear. Jews light a candle on the anniversary of a person's death to honor his or her memory. I am a WASP, so one day a year I pull out the heirlooms and set the table and honor the spirit of my mother this way.

This isn't a story about a mother whose kitchen emanated warmth and nurturing and inviting smells. It isn't a story about what an excellent cook my mother was, or how I learned to cook at her side. No, my mother's was a kitchen where pots banged and glass-paned cabinets slammed. My mother's was a kitchen where cooking dinner every night was a burdensome chore and getting my sister and me to eat it was worse. On a Saturday morning, if she was feeling ambitious, my mother might ask, "Would you like some pancakes?" If we said "sure," she'd slam a skillet and yell back, "For 'sure', I'm not making any pancakes! If you want pancakes, you can say 'yes, please.' Because I'm not cooking for 'sure.'"

My mother didn't like cooking for "sure" or for Monday, Tuesday, Wednesday, or Thursday. What my mother did like was entertaining. No one said "sure" at one of her parties. They said, "Yes, please, thank you, everything is wonderful." And it was.

My mother came late to cooking. Her mother, also short tempered, didn't allow her daughters in the kitchen while she cooked. My mother always resented that as a young woman in the '50s it was assumed she would know how to cook when she got married. Being ambitious, she applied herself diligently to mastering cookbooks and learned, but it was never natural, never instinctive, and never without a recipe. My father tells a story of my mother crying in the kitchen over a burnt beef stroganoff, while my father assured her that everyone was too drunk on martinis to know the difference.

In time she became a fabulous hostess. She said it all started when she couldn't get a babysitter for New Year's Eve the year I was born, so she just threw a party. It was also the first time my mother hadn't had a job since her teens, and I think that after my birth she felt she needed to keep challenging herself, if only in the kitchen. She had a wonderful group of friends to cook for: Mostly single, they all loved to eat and drink, and they were culinary adventurers who couldn't have cared less about calories or cholesterol. (Was there such a thing as cholesterol in 1965?) This crowd was the ideal audience; they praised her successes, devoured even her failures, and always arrived hungry.

Being a fabulous hostess requires both the ability to plan well and the talent and spontaneity to fly by the seat of one's pants. My mother was exceptional in both arenas. She could plan like a general and then, once the doorbell rang, let nature take its course. My mother had certain tenets of grand entertaining. First of all, she believed that everything should look lush and bountiful. Waste was not an issue in the entertainment universe of my mother, who believed that even when everyone had had his or her fill, there should be enough backup food in the kitchen to refill every serving dish on the buffet. Her second, and perhaps most important, belief was that there must always be enough alcohol. When I look back at what my mother spent on food versus drink, I realize why the party scene from *Breakfast at Tiffany's* is so familiar to me. My mother's parties often ended in the sort of innocent, lampshade-wearing drunkenness that hasn't been seen since the Beatles arrived in America. Lastly, my mother only befriended interesting and entertaining people. My husband always worries that I will invite over mismatched combinations of guests. This never occurs to me. I abide by my mother's belief that if all your friends are fun and interesting and have a lust for life, they will all naturally get along. Hers did, and mine do too.

I understand now why my mother loved to cook for parties and hated to cook us dinner. Maybe if she had kept her career she wouldn't have given a damn, but as it was, dinner was a big part of her day, and it seemed the harder she tried to cook something interesting, the more we hated it. In her cookbooks she has little notations about the family's response to certain dishes: *M & S: yes, Susan & Amanda: NO!*

Later in life, as years of martinis and chicken Cordon Bleu caught up with them, my mother's friends began to develop eating restrictions. These annoyed my mother, who considered them rude: "Pat has been so finicky since her bypass—won't even touch prosciutto. What a bore!" My mother would rather, and literally did, die before she limited what she ate. A cautious eater as a child, I now hear her voice ringing in my ears when I impulsively order the buffalo at Verbena because I want her to know I have grown up: Now I do want to experience life through my taste buds; I will not be narrow; I will try new things.

My mother died nine years ago. Two days before her death she asked my father to bring her a martini and a cigarette. When he brought the drink in a short tumbler she made him take it back and put it in her favorite stemmed glass. She sat in "her" chair and had one sip and one puff and returned to bed. The next day she asked my father to make her grits. I returned home from acting class to find my father's lumpy attempt congealing on the stove. The next morning she died. It seemed to me that she had traveled back through her taste buds: from the martinis of her single days in Manhattan in the '50s to the grits of her childhood in Arkansas.

So, now it is Christmas Eve and I am looking for the recipe for the lamb I am going to cook tomorrow. (The recipe is Greek, made with oodles of lemon juice and green beans that turn shriveled and black but squirt with the taste of lemon and lamb drippings when you bite into them.) I sit at my mother's kitchen table sifting through the boxes she kept her recipes in; these boxes are so old that they are cool again. The first is tin and has kitchen utensils painted on it in red, green, and black. The printed dividers (supplied with the box, a gift from *Good Housekeeping*) list categories such as "Meats & Savories," "The Henhouse," and "Sweets to the Sweet." I find the recipe I'm seeking under "Meats & Savories." Wondering what to serve with it, I turn to the other card file.

This box is milky green plastic, more '50s kitsch. This is where my favorite memories lie: This is where my mother kept her party menus. Thanksgiving dinners from 1968 until the '80s. Every dinner party, Christmas, New Year's Eve, and birthday dinner . . . the menus, the guest list, and sometimes the cost and a notation about what cookbook a particular dish was from. For example:

my mother's kitchen

February 1968—Theater Benefit

Shrimp Toast		
Kooftah Curry		
Rice Pilaf	Almaden Chablis	Food: $41.60
Tomato Aspic		Liquor: $62.29
Yogurt Cucumber		

·:·

I REMEMBER SHRIMP toast: It was a favorite appetizer of hers in the early '70s, when I was first old enough to help with the parties. I remember the pride of being part of the production, standing in the butler's pantry of our apartment, putting white paper doilies on large silver trays, my mother—in a maxi-length dress—pulling a cookie sheet of shrimp toast out of the oven. I held the tray conscientiously offering each person an hors d'oeuvre and a paper napkin. When they asked me what I was serving, I—in all my seven-year-old glory—would recite, "Shrimp Toast!" because I was in the know, because I had been in the kitchen with my mother.

It didn't take me long to become more involved in the kitchen. My mother's friend Brenda taught me to make baklava when I was twelve. My mother would schlep down to 9th Avenue, which used to be the Greek neighborhood, to buy me phyllo dough so I could bring baklava to the bake sale, while the other kids just brought brownies and chocolate chip cookies. I had inherited the show-off gene. It would drive my mother mad to see that they were charging the same twenty-five cents for my baklava as for everyone else's cookies. Still, it was the beginning of my entrepreneurship: Mrs. Finn, the math teacher, used to pay me ten dollars to make her baklava for Christmas, and I would swap a pan of baklava for a pecan pie from the Latin teacher, Mrs. Bennet.

I loved making baklava. It felt like a holiday each time I came home and found the ingredients my mother had bought for me, fresh and waiting on the counter top. Brenda had given me the cookbook in which she'd found her baklava recipe, and true to my mother's teaching, I wrote in the margin: *"Good, but a child needs a helper."* Not that I was a child, you understand. I was a competent cook. I pounded the walnuts with a meat mallet just as Brenda had shown me. I measured the dry ingredients carefully and watched the mixture of sugar, cinnamon, and walnuts transform beneath my spoon. I melted the butter, watching so it wouldn't burn, and then ever so carefully I spread out my phyllo sheets. The tricky part for me was lifting the sheets of pastry without tearing them. They were too big for the pan, so I painstakingly folded each one, alternating sides so that one side wouldn't be higher than the other. Once the pan was in the oven it was time to make the syrup: one cup honey, one cup sugar, one cup water with one teaspoon of orange juice. The syrup had to be timed just right so that you could pour it, simmering, over the baklava when it came out of the oven. You poured until it stopped sizzling. I always had leftover syrup, which I discovered was delicious on vanilla ice cream. Cooking absorbed me as few things had and my attention span increased in the kitchen. I was fearless. What greater reward for a twelve-year-old than the intense sweetness of a pastry made by her own hand?

After that, I became the family pastry chef, making desserts to complement my mother's dinners. Baklava remained my signature dish, but I also learned to make pumpkin pie, lemon pie, apple pie, buttermilk pie, almond bundt cake, pecan sandies, and bar cookies. After desserts I conquered pasta. There were definite periods: the dessert years, the pasta years, the salad years, the soup years. I'm currently in the meat years.

My mother became more ambitious as we got older. She took a Chinese cooking class, which culminated in an eight-course dinner cooked by the students, all women, for their husbands. My sister and

I loved anything cooked in the wok. As the '70s went on and the emphasis shifted to fresh vegetables and pasta, my sister and I began to love food. My mother would shop each afternoon for produce, bringing home such exotica as star fruit and kiwi. I'll never forget the thrill and the disappointment of the stalk of sugar cane she brought home. We used a saw to hack into it—only to discover it was stringy and tough—not sweet at all as I had imagined it would be.

I became even more of a help in my mother's kitchen. She could always rely on me to do some annoying task like grate Parmesan cheese or beat egg whites until stiff. When my aunt and uncle moved to the Midwest, we stopped spending Christmas at their home and my mother saw it as an opportunity to eliminate turkey from the holiday meal. That first year my mother decided to have an English Christmas: Roast beef, Yorkshire pudding, and trifle. I rallied behind the idea of internationally themed Christmases, and my mother and I would begin discussing our menu around Halloween. For a few years we went around the globe: lamb from Greece, goose with puréed chestnuts from Austria, and stuffed duckling and Champagne-pea soup from Denmark. Eventually we decided to stick with goose, but since my mother's death I have returned to the tradition of no tradition. I served salmon when my almost-vegetarian sister made it east from Montana, and revisited the Greek lamb of 1988 in 2000.

When crepes were all the rage my mother decided it would be fun to serve them at a party and let everyone fill their own. She had read that you could make crepes in advance and freeze them, so for two Saturdays before the big event my mother, my father, and I took turns making batter, ladling it into the special Teflon crepe pans, twisting to just coat, and flipping them out with a flick of the wrist—just before the edges got too dark. I can still remember her praising my technique. Was she just pulling a Tom Sawyer, flattering me into doing her "chores"? It doesn't matter—because

I love cooking. I love planning the menu—poring over old *Gourmet* magazines, my volumes of cookbooks, and clipped recipes. Unlike my mother, I love considering my audience: Are there any vegetarians, does someone really love a particular dish, are they spicy people, or creamy people? I relish the logistics of the time plot, balancing the ratio of top-of-stove items and inside-oven items as well as the cook-ahead items with those that must be prepared at the last minute. It thrills me to use every appliance my husband and I received for our wedding, and to set the table with our good china. As I heard my husband confide to another newly married man at one of our dinner parties, "At least she uses the stuff."

And yes, I love the food. After the intellectual work of planning, I hurl myself into the physicality of cooking. I abandon myself to the mess. There is nothing more grounding than digging my hands into a warm butternut squash and pulling out the seeds. Than the whirr of the blender as I purée it into the smoothest of soups. The challenge of boning my first duck in order to make my first *cassoulet* was terrifying, but as the hours slipped away and I began to understand the anatomy of a duck—there came the glory of hard-won knowledge, and ultimately the reward of a delectable *cassoulet*. What can compare to opening the oven door and seeing that yes, the chocolate soufflé did rise, just like the one in the picture? When I cook I am in the flow, time slips away, and worries fade.

Tomorrow, when the lamb is in the oven, when I am covered head to toe in flour, with watercress stems beneath my fingernails, I will clean the kitchen. I love to clean the kitchen. I love how my equipment comes up from the dishwater—shining and new. While the soup simmers and the cheese softens, I will slip into the shower and prepare to greet my guests. When I've put on a comfortable dress and the guests are around the table, I will relish that first sip of soup, and know, even before they tell me, that yes, it is good.

helen neottling's greek lamb

Surround leg of lamb in large roasting pan with whole green beans (you can trim the ends). Squeeze lemon juice over beans. Roast thirty minutes per pound at 300°, turning beans every thirty to forty-five minutes. Use one fistful of green beans per person and one lemon for every two people.

brenda mccauley's baklava

Pastry

1 cup sweet butter

2 cups chopped walnuts

¼ cup sugar

½ tsp. cinnamon

1 package phyllo dough

Syrup

1 cup honey

1 cup sugar

1 cup water

½ tsp. cinnamon

¼ tsp. salt

1 tsp. orange juice

Preheat oven to 350°.

Melt butter, spread on twelve phyllo sheets. Place sheets in buttered 11×14 *tin* pan. Mix nuts, sugar, and cinnamon together. Continue buttering phyllo sheets, one at a time, sprinkling each sheet with nut/sugar mixture. Butter remaining sheets and place on top. Cut pie into serving pieces. Bake for one hour.

Meanwhile, mix honey, sugar, water, cinnamon, salt, and orange juice together. Simmer fifteen minutes. Keep hot. Remove pastry from oven and pour hot honey mixture over. Stop pouring when sizzling stops (to avoid a sticky, gluey catastrophe). Cover, but do not refrigerate (this, too, seems to cause a sticky situation).

the art and science
of cocktail hour

{ R A C H E L   F U D G E }

İT'S A TUESDAY night in 1982. The sun has slipped
down far enough to bathe the concrete high-rises a block over in
a glorious shade of golden pink. Grabbing a handful of peanuts, I
nudge my mom, nearly spilling her vodka and tonic, and jerk my
head toward our neighbor across the street, who is clearly visible
through our plate-glass window and his uncurtained one. "It's the
underpants guy!" I chortle, as my brother turns his head away in
disapproval and focuses his attention on slicing perfect strips of
Gouda to accompany his stoned-wheat crackers. My dad sets his
drink down on a coaster and inquires, "Is the baby there, too?"
referring to our neighbor's habit of watching the evening news
while sprawled on his bed, clad only in boxer shorts and with his
small infant (who is usually clothed) nestled against his chest.
Perched atop one of San Francisco's biggest hills, our cozy flat isn't

big enough to afford much privacy, so it's a good thing that my parents and brother and I honestly enjoy one another's company.

·❖·

IT'S A THURSDAY night in 1992, and my junior paper—the thirty-page essay that's a core requirement for my history major—is due tomorrow. It's going to be a long night spent struggling with the economic, social, and political factors leading up to the 1904 Chicago meatpackers' strike, but right now, as I nurse my second (and last) gin fizz of the evening, I haven't a care in the world. At the other end of the once-grand leather sofa, my pals Jane and Tim are gossiping about the cute new sophomore boys. From our vantage point in the middle of the living room, we can survey all the goings-on in the shabby-chic Tudor mansion we call home. Before long, the Bettie Serveert album that's been playing all week will drive me crazy, but now it still sounds perfect: with the drinks, my friends, and the music, nothing could be better. My parents are three thousand miles away and I miss them terribly, but I'm also utterly, improbably, at home here in New Jersey.

·❖·

IT'S A WEDNESDAY night in 2002, and the fog that has already engulfed the rest of the city hasn't yet closed in on my sunbelt neighborhood. It's really too chilly to sit outside, but we can't resist making the most of this still-clear evening, so I grab our jackets as Hugh finishes mixing up a small batch of martinis. Huddled on a deck chair, I start spreading cheap (but eminently edible) Brie on the remnants of yesterday's baguette, while Hugh has a one-sided chat with the skittish little black cat who divides his time between our neighbor's lush, well-tended garden and our own rickety, second-story deck. Pushing aside thoughts of dinner prep and imminent car repairs, we slowly sip our drinks and ponder our neighbor's landscaping choices *(What good is an eight-by-eight-foot patch of lawn? If you went to all the trouble of having a hot tub craned over the top of the house and installed in the backyard, wouldn't you spring for a material other than woodgrain-imprinted plastic?).* Hugh has a big deadline so he has to go back to the office after dinner, and I have to spend the evening figuring out my self-employment taxes, but for the next twenty minutes or so none of that matters.

⁘

FOR AS LONG as I can remember, my parents have practiced a once noble middle-class tradition turned dying art: the cocktail hour. Every evening, after my parents came home from work, changed their shoes, and washed their faces, my family would gather in the kitchen, where my parents would mix drinks and my brother and I would assemble the all-important snack tray of cheese and crackers, olives, peanuts, or chips and salsa. We'd all retire to the living room for a half-hour or so of casual conversation, trying to keep the *Brady Bunch* plot descriptions to a minimum. After consuming an almost-dinner-ruining amount of cheese or peanuts, my brother and I might get bored and disappear to our bedrooms, leaving my parents to a few precious minutes of sanity, postponing dinner preparation, homework help, and bill paying.

This family ritual has endured for decades, with only slight changes in timing, cast of characters, and vittles. Certain key factors persist, however: Everyone takes a moment to sit down together, the TV stays off, behavior remains civil (in other words, the tantrums are reserved for after dinner). Pacing and consistency are the key elements here—not the gin. Family friends and acquaintances may have been slightly alarmed to hear my brother and me extol the virtues of "cocktails," but in our minds, "having cocktails" really meant early-evening family snacktime. (It wasn't until I got to college that I began to understand just how soothing that pre-dinner alcoholic beverage could be.) Cocktail hour wasn't only about the booze, though my parents certainly enjoyed their drinks; it was also about decompression and transition, an informal but nonetheless reliable moment of family togetherness.

These days it's difficult to champion alcoholic beverages of any kind, not least cocktails, without sending up warning signals of excess. The 1990s' resurrection of cocktail culture (swing bands, swank bars, and bastardized martinis) focused on re-creating the seemingly more civilized drinking atmosphere of years gone by, yet it's clear as ice-cold vodka that those days of yore were hardly as halcyon as contemporary cocktail mythology would have us believe. While some of my peers continue to aestheticize the drinking habits of their parents and grandparents, others are desperately trying to recover from them.

This is nothing new, of course; as long as there's been drink, there've been drunks. But reading coming-of-age tales set in the 1960s and '70s, you'd think that everyone's parents invited the neighbors over for a pre-dinner cocktail that inevitably turned into an extended binge, with dinner long forgotten and adults turned giddy and untrustworthy, even menacing. Those aren't the only narratives, however. For some families—my own unabashedly included—cocktails are a regenerative, not destructive, force.

The cocktail hour is, in my opinion, a secret ingredient in an enduring relationship, and the cornerstone of drinking's socializing effect. My parents, who recently celebrated their thirty-fifth wedding anniversary, are a testament to its rejuvenative power. One could say that I am the progeny of the cocktail, because in fact both sets of my grandparents were married for more than fifty years. And now I seem to be continuing that tradition myself: My partner, Hugh, and I are heading toward our tenth year together—no small feat for a couple who only just hit thirty. I can't lay all the credit with the cocktail hour, but I can say for certain that "It's six o'clock; the bar's open" was a familiar refrain in my grandparents' and my parents' homes. I wouldn't go so far as to say that the family that drinks together stays together, but I do think the ritual celebration of the cocktail can help anchor a stable, happy, and communicative home life.

Lest I imply otherwise, my family is not composed of especially heavy or single-minded drinkers. The rituals of drinking—icing the glasses and carefully stirring the martinis in homage to my dad's father, who enjoyed his with an extra olive and promptly at 6:00 P.M.; laying out the cheese board and slicer—are as exhilarating as alcohol's heady effects. When, on special occasions, my dad can be cajoled into blending a batch of whisky sours, it isn't so much the actual drink that I adore (though I do love it); it's the comforting taste of history, of those silly yet unassailable family traditions whose origins no one can remember—like shooting hoops on Christmas Eve and cheerfully suffering through frigid and fogged-in Fourth of July barbecues. A bite of a madeleine transports Proust into reflective and verbose bliss; gin and tonics and extra-sharp cheddar are all that are needed to send me on a lengthy nostalgia trip.

This sentiment of sociability and ritual grace has resonated throughout my extrafamilial drinking life. Upon my arrival at the hallowed halls of a certain Ivy League university well known for its history of inebriated gentility, I was nearly swept away by the sea of tepid, unredeemable beer served in sticky-floored basements. Fortunately, I escaped the wave of Meister Brau before any liver damage was done, and I soon reverted to the more civilized forms of drinking with which I'd grown up. I had the great fortune to eat, drink, and socialize in a house where food was love, and drink enhanced the most sumptuous aspects of any menu. Balancing indulgence with temperance—these were the keys to happy, healthy living as espoused by our chef and ringleader, who craftily introduced persnickety college students to the delights of both the ever-healthful broccoli rabe and the headily decadent Death by Chocolate Cake. One of the mainstays of the house rituals was the pre-dinner cocktail hour on Thursdays, a weekly event that got many of us through the travails of midterms, senior theses, love affairs, and sundry personal crises. It was in college that I learned there are few things more glorious or comforting in life than sitting on a sun-warmed stoop with one's best friends, sipping a vodka gimlet, dissecting the subtext of that week's *Beverly Hills, 90210*, and watching the sun set below the trees.

In the first years after graduation, it was more difficult to maintain the regular cocktail hour. While Hugh and I were eager to settle into homebound domesticity (not to mention eager to avoid shelling out our hard-earned dollars for watered-down drinks in overcrowded bars), many of our friends and coworkers were more enamored of the cocktail hour's arch-nemesis, the *happy* hour. If one is single, or living alone, it becomes necessary to go out for a drink, rather than stay in—especially if one upholds the first caveat of cocktail hour: togetherness. But rather than settling for "happy hour," that rather grim invention created by bars to get folks in and imbibing as early as possible, I preferred to host my own cocktail hours.

Now, some will argue in favor of the cocktail party, that admittedly more debaucherous gathering. A good cocktail party is an underappreciated social art these days, but its properties are decidedly different: Unlike cocktail hour, which is at heart about insularity and introspection, the cocktail party is for the extrovert. The cocktail hour isn't about ostentation, flirtatious double entendres, or knowing which impossibly hip drink to order. In fact, it's the exact opposite: domestic comfort, routine, and a complete lack of pretense.

Besides, a key ingredient in the cocktail hour is domesticity, thus requiring a private rather than a public venue. The underlying function of the cocktail hour is to create a smooth transition from work to relaxation, from hectic to tranquil. It's about arriving home from work (in my case, shutting down the computer and heading upstairs from my basement office when I hear Hugh come in the front door), kicking off my shoes, putting dinner plans and the day's mail on hold, and rustling up a drink, even if it's only a glass of cheap Australian Syrah. It's about slapping a favorite LP on the turntable (blues-inflected punk rock goes very well with cocktails), slumping on the couch or perching on the back deck, and chatting about absolutely nothing of consequence. Drink in hand, loved one at my side, this is the essence of home.

classic martini

AS PREPARED BY THREE GENERATIONS OF
THE FUDGE FAMILY

Cocktail shaker

Double-ended jigger

Gin (at room temperature)

Dry vermouth

Green olives

Set two martini glasses in the freezer to chill. Fill the cocktail shaker half-full of ice cubes. Measure out two large jiggers (about 4 oz.) of gin and 1 small jigger (½ oz.) of vermouth. Shake vigorously. Add two olives to each chilled glass. Pour martini over olives. Reserve any leftover liquid for dividends. For a dirty martini, add a splash of olive juice. Serves two.

nurturing the tough guy

{ JOSIE AARONSON-GELB }

AFTER MOVING TO a town in a strange state with no friends to speak of, I fleshed out my one-woman social circle with a rumor that flamed like cognac in a pan: *Have you met the new gal? Man, can she cook.* No one had ever tasted my food. Ever. All it took to get a reputation of culinary genius was to *talk* about food, describe favorite spices, shop competently at Albertson's, and sometimes, with a few casual mentions in getting-to-know-you conversation, drop information about past restaurant work experience. Add to that a wine and cheese gathering I hosted in order to showcase a quarter pound of Humboldt Fog with a finger of blue snaking through it like a single vein, and my reputation was made.

The truth is, the twenty-something generation is so lost in the kitchen that anyone who can wield a spatula, or even talk about a spatula, holds unparalleled power. As it stands right now I am a voodoo doctor—a strange and mysterious being capable of transforming raw garlic into a roasted spread. Magician-like, I can simmer lentil soup in thirty minutes and sear tuna in five. The mere promise of culinary sizzle brings new friends out of the woodwork with chants of praise and worship—people from the convenience-foods generation, people for whom cooking from scratch is a minor miracle, lost souls who moved out of their parents' houses and started cooking for themselves in a decade when instant meals—those microwavable, dehydrated, canned, and pre-made gems—had roots firmly planted in every aisle of every grocery store across the country.

Why bother to shop for bean sprouts, cilantro, lime, fish sauce, and peanuts, when instant *pad thai* noodles are available for ninety-nine cents a cellophane-wrapped pop? Why delve into the wild world of enchiladas when you can buy them frozen, with organic beans, for $2.99, and forgo all that chopping, seasoning, filling, wrapping, and baking? I'm not trying to imply that twenty-somethings are lazy, it's just that we're living in an era of shortcuts: You can microwave for two minutes or work for twenty, risk your vegetables rotting before you find time to use them or shop in the freezer section for those nice little compartments of peas sitting alongside frozen lumps of chicken Parmesan. And, of course, all of those pre-packaged meals come with exact calorie counts and nutritional breakdowns; people who shop pre-packaged can chart every dollop of fat that goes into their bodies.

For this reason, perhaps, it is women who are most often enthu-siastic about the idea of home-cooked meals but, when it comes down to the actual cooking, pale at the prospect of preparation. It takes age and a certain *je ne sais quoi* for many women to rid them-selves of food phobia and culinary reluctance. To live in a house where you actually keep more than one kind of oil on hand (the fat! the calories!) is to live in an alternate universe. On my shelf there is a burnt red bottle of chili oil; nutty, dark liquid sesame;

plain-Jane canola; and, my pride and joy, a deep sea-green olive oil imported from Italy and bitter like I imagine uncured olives to be.

When I am in the kitchen with a new guest, a culinary virgin, I try to trick her into turning her back before the oil or butter goes into any dish—a ruse left over from my time cooking in the restaurant industry. In professional kitchens fat is used to enhance flavor, to smooth out sauces, to crisp edges. In professional kitchens, fat is nothing to be afraid of. But in the outside world, even the strongest women I know are shocked by it. Lara, a die-hard feminist lit student who uses "she" as the *only* subject pronoun and thinks that women who let their boyfriends encircle their waists in public are selling out to patriarchy, nearly fainted in her running shoes when she witnessed my treatment of sautéed potatoes, paling as the lump of butter collapsed in the pan, meandering around the hot silver circle in a pool of its own languidity. Her eyes widened when I added to that pale butter a quarter cup of olive oil, the two fats swirling together, foaming. I won her over in the end. I dare you to show me the person who can remain empty-stomached in a kitchen as it fills up with the nutty smell of caramelizing onions and garlic, the promising pop of potatoes—just don't let them watch you cook.

Not that I'm a total stranger to the fear of fat. When I was in school studying restaurant management, tucked into my chef's outfit in the test kitchens, I poured warm cream into hot roux, added pounds of Fontina cheese, and didn't taste it once. Yes, I wanted to own a restaurant. Yes, I wanted to be a super-star chef. But I wanted to do it as a five-foot-three-inch barrel of female power standing on a step stool to reach the eggs on the top shelf of the walk-in refrigerator. I wanted to be the delicate little miss bossing great galumphing men around with a wag of her weightless hips.

The professional kitchen is still a man's world and the idea that to fit into it a female chef must be a hulking, I'll-take-anything-you-throw-at-me, wanna-arm-wrestle kind of person makes me crazy. Of course, fighting this man-chef image is not about eating cabbage soup until your pants fall off, but resisting internalized notions of femininity and masculinity. In the professional kitchen, being female, being *womanly,* is something to keep hidden. It is much more common to find women who look and sound as rugged and tough as the guys than to find the nurturing type, sugar and spice and everything nice. The few times I've worked with other women in professional kitchens, they have, on the outside, been the most hardened of the bunch.

In the restaurant kitchen there is an initial intense rivalry between the women behind the stovetop. I have yet to work in a kitchen where the women on staff (never more than two) welcome me with open arms. This isn't true in the other professions in which I've worked. In fact, in all business environments, regular nine-to-five worlds revolving around tiny cubicles and one-page memos, the bonding between female coworkers has been touchy-feely, lets-share-lives-and-go-get-salads-for-lunch kind of action. Not in the kitchen.

I have a theory about why. A new woman who enters the kitchen and likes to talk about relationships and analyze interpersonal dynamics, who doesn't make sexual remarks about the wait staff (about the way they look, dress, flirt), might remind the male workers that *Oh my god, women exist in the work environment! They are right here next to us, slinging spinach more efficiently than we do, deglazing roasting pans with more skill. Alert, alert, a woman is getting the better of me! I. Must. Fight. Back.* And so—*boom!*—there goes the chummy relationship that the first woman, the original tough-guy cook, had with her male coworkers. Women in the kitchen need to act tough to counter the fact that they are women. Because once they are considered—*gasp*—female, the dynamic of the kitchen is disrupted.

Sexual competition behind the line is part of any new woman's entry into a restaurant. But that woman will never fit into the team atmosphere until she can negate her femininity and establish that she is more than a potential date. It is only after this occurs that she will be viewed as someone who can be relied on and trusted to do her job without spurring flirtatious competition, and therefore friction, among her male coworkers. I have never worked in a restaurant where the male chefs didn't treat me like a piece of meat, a potential girlfriend, a hook-up, until I proved that I could cuss with the best of them, sling food in a pan with the strongest of them, and make disparaging comments about the female wait staff too.

Part of the machismo that flows through professional kitchens can be attributed directly to the gender division between front- and back-of-house staff. While not always the case, the general breakdown in any upscale American restaurant kitchen is women out front, men in back. There is a huge disparity in both appearance and action between these two intertwined professions. Working in the front of house is an intensely psychological and mentally challenging game. The serving staff, the front-of-house beauties, are generally thin and pretty, with made-up faces and a paycheck that often relies on subdued (or blatant) flirtation. They keep clean, and are polite and friendly in order to score the biggest tips.

The back-of-house cooks play in a different world entirely. Hidden behind impenetrable kitchen doors, they have no need to be either well groomed or well behaved. Professional kitchen staff members are measured in terms of *my grill flame is bigger than your grill flame*, or *I bet I can flip more onions, in a heavier skillet, than you*. When the serving staff come in, clean and proper and lipsticked, to check on orders prepared by the sweating, food splattered cooks, it is no wonder the tension is so heavy. After all, the cooks are *working*. They're *sweating*. They're being *men*. And those front-of-house chicks, all they have to do is refill wine and smile, right? Wrong, as any waitress will tell you. The wait staff have a difficult job in that they field guest complaints, have to apologize for kitchen blunders, and smooth things over if a guest is unhappy. Of course, they also get all the pleasure of accepting compliments for a meal well prepared, for timing perfectly executed. The kitchen does not. Maybe the head chef gets written up in the newspaper but the line cooks, the sous-chef, everyone else working hot, steamy hours in the back of the house goes unrecognized.

I remember one week when I was working behind the line with Evan, the grill man who, after I refused to go out with him and made fun of his mother a little bit, made an excellent ally. While working his own station he was also helping me fry up made-to-order *fritto misto*—paper thin lemon slices, baby artichokes, and calamari—when we were slammed. While he was working, juggling some of my orders and all of his, a ceramic ramekin fell into the vat of oil he stood over and sent a splash of boiling grease up over his exposed wrist and hand. Without even pausing, he wrapped the burn in a water-soaked towel and kept working. When the towel dried out he removed it, and for the rest of the four-hour shift, held his injured arm directly over foot-long flames while he continued to broil close to thirty steaks an hour. The next day he came to work with a mass of fluid-filled bubbles marking his arm.

Scarred and burned arms are part of the cook's job, just like a nail through the thumb might be for a carpenter, or migraines for a teacher. Trying to keep up with this industry-wide *pain, what pain?* attitude has gotten me more permanent scars than any of the men I have ever worked with.

When I ran a kitchen near Yosemite National Park in California, my co-manager was a man who liked to lift things and take things out of the top oven for me. This, remember, is the ultimate professional crime, being recognized as smaller or weaker or female. I was worried that my authority would be undermined if I couldn't remove the baby-bathtub-sized metal pan holding still-bubbling baked beans from the oven by myself. I ended up with calf burns. Or, when I couldn't find a milk crate to use as a stepping stool, I removed the bacon from the top oven anyway, spilling hot grease on my arms. Still, I responded to all offers of help with firm, sarcastic refusals.

In the kitchen there is no excuse for being injured, sick, or in emotional crisis. Whatever you're feeling, you hide it and continue to sear meat, dice leeks, sauté pancetta with asparagus, and push through. To back away from a challenge, to take the easy way out—whether that be calling in sick when you have pneumonia, or a heat-sensitive rash up and down your arms—spells doom for the professional chef. Yes, taste buds and a sense of flavor combinations are important, but more important are endurance and a suck-it-up mentality.

This is precisely what angers me about professional kitchens—this idea that in order to fit in you have to get respect the way football players do, through brutishness. In one kitchen I shared a shift with Janet. She was a large woman, a garbage-mouthed line cook who was cruder to the waitresses than any of the men. She used the word "bitch" like a piece of punctuation and got pissed off when I wore eyeliner to work. One day she came into work late. Her best friend had just had a baby and she had been there for the birth. It surprised me to think of Janet, the tough slur-tossing cook, having female friends, not to mention participating in an intimate, emotional, and wholly womanly occurrence. After that day, I studied her to see how she stayed so strong and impenetrable, and, well, masculine, for ten hours a day, five to six days a week, when I knew there was a softer side to her.

I never saw her cave. Her sarcasm toward me diminished only when I proved I could handle a slamming two hours of non-stop orders, only when I poured a half-cup of oil into a single pan without cringing, only when I stopped wearing makeup. Only then did she start speaking to me, and even then only in a how-'bout-those-49ers manner. All I can figure is that she kept her private life out of the kitchen, that she understood the rules of the game and was willing to play. I wasn't.

This is the difference between women who cook at home and women who cook professionally. Historically, for home chefs, food has been about nurturing, feeding the family, expressing love, and caretaking. I love this part of cooking. I love inviting friends into my house, sitting them down and making them feel relaxed and at home, even when their real families are miles away.

Perhaps this gender divide between professional and home cooking is why it is difficult for twenty-something American women—women raised as freethinking, feminist-minded, career-oriented people—to find a good balance in their relationship with food. The new generation of men is caught in a similar predicament. For years, most of their mothers handled the food for the whole family. Even in the '80s and '90s, the realm of home cooking still belonged to women. My male friends each have one—two if they've had a girlfriend who taught them something—dish that they make for dinner. I make it a point to look in cupboards and refrigerators when I go over to their houses. What I find shocks me: Bread. Eggs (maybe). Peanut butter. Salt. Pepper. Frozen potatoes. There are no herbs. There are no vegetables. There is no cooking.

So, because modern women have been fighting to stay out of the home kitchen, and men have yet to pick up the slack and learn the craft of home cooking, there is an entire generation of people who have no love for the creation of food. These are people who are hunting for mates, who are concerned about health and shun the fast food gobbled up by the majority of America's youth. But these are also people who could not feed themselves if all the frozen-food packaging plants, restaurants, and canneries suddenly closed down.

And this is why I wow them. I admit, I love to wow my friends.

There is nothing I enjoy more than gathering a group of people around a dish full of citrus tomatillo enchiladas, a plate of sautéed sweet peppers and corn, some lime-zest sour cream, and watching them dig in. They are all polite; manners are still something that they know. They all *ooh* and *aah* and I love the attention. I can't deny it. But I would trade all of that for a crowd of friends who could cook with me. Who wouldn't close their eyes and shriek at the sight of oil. For a professional kitchen where the competition isn't in who can toss the penne the highest, but who can forge the strongest friendships, who can crack the divide that separates men and women, meld the rift between front of house and back of house, on the shift. As it stands right now, the fate of food and cooking is in social limbo. Men are not stepping up to the plate at home, and women are only slowly stepping up to the professional one, and only in disguise.

Sometimes, especially when I am cooking for men, I worry that in the hiss of my pan, in the steam from the oven, I am expressing too many old-fashioned tendencies. I get paranoid that I am acting too motherly to be taken seriously as a swinging single. When that happens, I choke mid-bite, mid-compliment, and start to downplay my love for cooking, or worse, defend it by showcasing my rough and tumble burns from working in professional kitchens. But then I remember: Food is my skill, and it is a shareable one. That's not old-fashioned, or socially backward, it's just my way of expressing friendship. And if I can slip in a little extra fat to amp up the flavor without anyone freaking out, well, I'll consider myself lucky. After all, they do it in restaurants all the time.

baking boot camp

{ LISA JERVIS }

SUNDAY

THE WEEK I'VE been looking forward to for the past six months is finally here: Baking Boot Camp at the Culinary Institute of America, in Hyde Park, New York. It's a thirtieth birthday gift from my parents and the culmination of years of baking hobbyism that, in the last year or so, has become quite an obsession.

One day I stumbled across information about what seemed to be the perfect vacation: a five-day intensive course for nonprofessional "food enthusiasts" that combines instruction with some serious eating. For the next week, I will bake all day and then dine once at each of the CIA's swanky restaurants. I'm ready for intense food-science information and yummy baked goods.

After checking into the dorm, I head over to orientation. A man with a clipboard hands me an ugly miniduffel filled with goodies and points the way to a small auditorium-style classroom. They said there would be food at this thang, and I'm disappointed to find only a small platter of cheese and crackers and some nuts. I haven't eaten since 11:00 A.M. and was hoping for something more substantial. I get myself a plate and take a seat next to a very friendly woman named Franny, who, it turns out, is in my class. After I figure out that my desk slides out of the arm of the chair in a deceptively simple way, Franny needs to get out. I think I can just get up with my tray still extended. Ha! I send my drink flying and the plate to the ground. CIA employees rush to my aid. I'm too embarrassed to replace my snack.

I check out the contents of my bag: a uniform (the pants are as ugly as I feared) and my kit (an ingenious little bag that rolls up and snaps closed, containing some knives, a peeler, a couple scrapers, various other tools, and—just what I've always wanted—my very own offset spatula). There's also a CIA-branded binder containing the course curriculum and recipes. Tomorrow's lesson is the creaming method. According to my manual, by the end of the next day I should be able to describe how to repair a creaming-method batter that has separated. Wheee! Maybe I'll also learn why my chocolate chip cookies always come out totally flat and wrinkly.

After orientation, I learn a bit about my fellow students over burgers at the snack bar. Jenn just quit her job as a computer programmer to do an eighteen-month baking and pastry program. This week is her test to make sure that a year and a half of baking is what she really wants to do. Dana, who's here for one of the CIA's continuing-education courses for food professionals, cooks for a midwestern sports team–owning family. She's enrolled in Artisan Breads. I'm jealous. Bread has been my big preoccupation ever since I determined to get over my fear of yeast. I've gotten some decent results at home, but nothing with the open texture and chewy crust I crave. I would definitely forgo croissants and puff pastry for baguettes, bagels, and old-school Jewish rye. On the other hand, I'm grateful I won't see Dana every day after she cautions me not to eat too much this week, and patronizingly pronounces the boot camp curriculum and tools "too baby" for her.

I get in bed with my sleazy mystery novel and fall asleep early in preparation for waking up at 5:15. Not for the first time, I wonder why I have chosen a vacation that requires me to rise before dawn.

MONDAY

A.M.

THE SUN'S NOT even up when I arrive at breakfast. The Breakfast Cookery students have been here for hours, preparing to serve things like poached eggs with chicken à la King, a farmer's omelet, and cornmeal waffles with caramel sauce and strawberries. I don't usually eat so soon after waking, and the hour makes me a little nauseated. But I know if I don't get some food in me I'll never stay awake. Plus, well, when else will I get the chance to eat like this without waiting an hour for a table at a precious, overpriced brunch eatery at home? I get the waffle—it's good, but it doesn't sit quite right, and I decide that for the rest of the week my breakfast will be plain poached eggs on toast (although one day later in the week I choose Cream of Wheat, which seems to be made with actual cream).

There are eleven of us in this little classroom, eyeing each other curiously as we pull at our ill-fitting, stiff uniforms. Who in their right mind designs chef's pants to run so small? At least two of my classmates can't even wear theirs. I go through the week with only the bottom two snaps on my fly buttoned.

Our instructor, Chef Henry, arrives at the stroke of the hour, sporting a neatly trimmed mustache and a militarily precise demeanor. He's doubtless a total hardass with the real students, but I can tell he's going to treat us a little more gently. We go around the room and introduce ourselves. In addition to me, Jenn, and

Franny, we've got Maureen, an early-forties, smarty-pants management consultant from New Jersey; Lily and Fred, a father-daughter
team, which is very sweet and makes me wonder if my mother
would ever take a vacation that requires her to wake up before 6:00
A.M.; Katherine, who runs a small bakery in Massachusetts; George,
recently retired from the phone company, whose ambition is to perfect his deeply flawed apple pie; Will and Ted, air force enlistees
whose job it is to cook for four-star generals (they come to be known
as the flyboys); and Derrick, who runs a high-tech business and,
because I sit down next to him, becomes my partner for the week.

Chef Henry gives us a quick rundown of the creaming method—
it's news to me that when you add eggs to cookie batter, you're making an emulsion—then parcels out assignments. Derrick and I will
make pumpkin bread and oatmeal fruit cookies. We head downstairs
to get acquainted with the bakeshop and scale out the ingredients
for the day's production. Derrick and I manage to cooperate just
enough to get our batters mixed and the breads in the oven. Everything takes twice as long as it would have if I'd been on my own:
Derrick seems to be more interested in trying to impress the chef
with his questions about what oven techniques to use for bread than
actually, say, baking something. He combines the worst elements of
a science nerd personality (tossing around technical terms; assuring
me that math is his "thing" when I ask him if he is sure a meas-
urement is correct) with status-and-money-obsessed dot-com arrogance. He talks a lot about very expensive cookware and uses his
cell phone to check his stock portfolio while I clean up our station.
I don't think he cares for me too much either, but I don't give a shit.

P.M.

AFTER WE INSPECT and sample the morning's quick breads
(banana, date nut, Derrick's and my pumpkin—in which the

chocolate chips have sunk disappointingly to the bottom—and several pound cakes with various amounts of chemical leaveners so we can see and taste the differences), Chef Henry makes the perfect pie crust before our very eyes. It's a revelation. Turns out I've been scared off the proper technique by all those cookbooks that threaten doom by gluten for doughs with more than three drops of water and five seconds of mixing. Chef used about twice as much water, and worked the dough about twice as long, as I have always thought proper. And it's so springy! It feels soft and resilient at the same time. Gorgeous. Now that I have a sense memory of quality pie dough, I may venture past cakes and cookies more often.

❖

I'M SHOCKED AT how hungry I am by the time dinner rolls around. I feel like I've been eating all day, but by a quarter to six I'm ready to faint. Tonight we eat at St. Andrew's, the health-conscious restaurant on campus. This is the first time I experience wine carefully matched to food. While I do not plan to become a wine snob, I'm fascinated by the way a sweet wine suddenly tastes not sweet at all when sipped after a mouthful of cherries and sweet onions.

TUESDAY

A.M.

IT'S THE RUBBED method today: scones, biscuits, pie dough. Derrick and I are assigned a variation on the standard biscuit; we're adding cheddar, jalapeños, scallions, and pimentos. I am a little intimidated at first because I have some, um, issues with rolling, and the biscuit method is all about rolling. You barely mix the dry and wet ingredients into a shaggy mass, and then roll it out, fold it into thirds, roll again, and repeat. So the rolling is the way the dough comes together in the first place. But it isn't hard at all—very forgiving—and Derrick pretty much lets me do it all.

Or maybe I bulldoze him. He's surprisingly not confident in the kitchen. It seems strange that someone who would choose to vacation in a bakeshop would have so little intuition about it all. He can't proceed without having the chef check almost everything ("Is this a shaggy mass?"), and later, when we're mixing up our Danish dough (a project that will take three days to go from ingredients to finished pastry), he uses his digital watch to time two minutes at low speed and four at medium. What happened to just sticking your finger in there and feeling the damn thing? That's what makes it fun to bake in the first place, and I do not appreciate being told, when I know the dough is ready, that there are still seventeen seconds to go.

P.M.

AFTER LUNCH WE'VE all finished our morning assignment and done the first step in tomorrow's work, in my case the aforementioned Danish; for others puff pastry and croissants. So we bake off some of the cookies from yesterday. Everyone's production lined up on the counter looks beautiful: blueberry scones, the most uniform chocolate chip cookies ever, some Death by Chocolate cookies that for some reason refused to spread properly. And, of course, the cheese-scallion-pepper-pimento biscuits. I am proud.

After we all taste the various goodies, Chef gives us a little primer on yeast. I get the chance to see, touch, and taste fresh yeast for the first time. It looks a lot like the modeling clay I built a castle out of in my sixth-grade social studies class. Tastes strong, beery, a little musty. *Mm-mmm.* Chef sings its praises, but given how hard it is for the nonprofessional to find a reliable source, I think I'll stay away. And instant yeast seems like nothing special so far as I can tell. So, you don't have to put it in liquid before you add it to your thang. Big honkin' deal. I'll keep buying super-cheap active dry yeast from the bulk bins at Berkeley Bowl.

Next is what I've really come for. In preparation for our class, Chef Henry borrowed a bit of sourdough starter from a friend and has been feeding it since last Friday. We'll use it on the last day of class. I can't wait. It smells fantastic, just like a good loaf of bread. It's a lot drier than the starter I had going six months ago, which produced several batches of failed bread. (At first it tasted sour but never rose; when I helped it along with some added commercial yeast, it wiped out all the lovely sour flavor.) I learn that (contrary to the recipe I had been using) it's better to avoid putting whole-grain flours in a starter because the oils can go rancid. Are rancid and moldy the same thing? I gave up on my starter when some mold appeared around the rim of the bowl.

My classmates and I attend a coffee and tea tasting. Our instructor, Isabella Grimshaw, is very frazzled. I picture the culinary school equivalent of nasty office politics, with chef-instructors raiding each other's caches of *foie gras* and whispering about a persistent burnt flavor in their rivals' brown roux. As soon as we get down to the dining room to begin the actual tasting, though, a competent calm descends and her slightly daft passion for hot beverages comes through. She is unable to contain her excitement as she unfurls tea leaves in the palm of her hand and passes them around so we can examine their shape. She speaks with scorn of those who refer to "herbal tea," and I learn that there is no such thing: All true tea comes from a plant called *Camellia sinensis*, and all those things we know as herbal tea are accurately called herbal infusions. She looks like a benevolent mad genius, in her glasses and lab coat. I feel myself developing an enormous crush on her.

In spite of my fear of drinking too much caffeine, I can't resist the chance to compare and contrast Sumatran light roast, Sumatran dark roast, Kenyan, Costa Rican, and two different versions of the same Colombian, one roasted just the other day and one roasted who knows how long ago. The big surprise: The biggest difference is between the two Colombians—the same exact beans. I'll be buying my coffee in tiny batches in the future.

Afterward, I head over to the library to watch *Bread and Baker: From the Source, Part 3* and something called *Power of Flour.* I learn to tell the difference between bread, cake, and pastry flours by look and feel. I can't take notes fast enough, there's so much information I want to absorb: ideal temperatures for starter, fermentation-promoting minerals in rye . . . I embrace my inner bread geek: Can I buy these videos in the bookstore?

·❖·

THE CLASS RENDEZVOUS at Caterina de' Medici, the campus Italian restaurant, where we eat what turns out to be far and away the best dish of the week: cavatelli with wild mushrooms and thyme. The waiter tells us that the pasta is flown in from Italy, frozen rather than dried, at a cost of six dollars a pound. That last bit is annoying—do I really care?—but it cannot diminish my pleasure. The lamb chops that follow are excellent but anticlimactic. Dessert is not very appealing—some kind of fruit-embedded cake—and for this I am thankful, since in the past two days I feel like I have eaten four days' worth of food. It's a good group, everyone's friendly, and we seem to be finding plenty of innocuous things to talk about—until the cake is served and someone starts talking about Iraq. The topic spreads from one table to the other so that suddenly we're all discussing it. I'm sitting next to George, whose moderate views will luckily not bring us to blows.

Shockingly, it turns out that I agree most with Maureen, who describes herself as a conservative Republican. We segue into a discussion of feminism and fiscal conservatism versus social conservatism.

I'm very glad I'm not at the table with the flyboys, who have so antagonized die-hard Democrat Franny that she seems near tears. As we leave the restaurant, Will cheerfully exclaims "Vote Bush!" as a tongue-in-cheek but nonetheless quite hostile goodnight.

WEDNESDAY

A.M.

DERRICK AND I struggle for four hours to get through the process of laminating our Danish dough. It is as hard and frustrating as I had expected, but still fun. First we roll the dough (which has been chilling in the walk-in overnight) into a rectangle. The easy part ends there. Then we take our three pounds—what seems like a huge amount—of butter and hit it with a rolling pin to make it pliable.

We need to roll this mound of butter out into a thick, even sheet half the size of the dough rectangle, while not letting it get too warm and melty. It's supposed to be the same firmness as the dough itself, so that when the two are rolled together everything will be even. Oh, lordy.

We form some sort of approximate butter-rectangle and get it "locked into" the dough, i.e., placed on top of half the dough with the other half folded over it so it's completely enclosed (or, in other words, laminated). Then we chill the dough some more, roll it out thin again, and fold it over to create all those alternating layers of dough and butter that will make it flaky and gorgeous—if we don't tear the dough, let the butter get too warm and squish out, or let any of the other things that can ruin it happen.

Of course, we won't really know how good a job we've done until we bake the pastries on Friday. But the lamination feels successful. I have my first glimmer of good rolling technique. "Become one with the pin," advises Chef Henry. "Also, relax," he adds.

Mmm-kay! That is clearly the key, but can I alter my essential personality to become a better baker?

Today's workload is pretty light, so there's time to stand around, look over other people's shoulders, and ask nonessential questions. I enjoy the pace, which confirms for me that I never want to be more than a highly skilled hobbyist in the kitchen. I watch as Jenn rolls the most gorgeous batch of croissant dough. It has edges like a ruler. I am jealous. I started out saying that I would never laminate dough at home, but now I'm imagining my friends *oohing* and *aahing* over homemade Danish and croissants.

NOON

AFTER LUNCH CHEF bows to popular demand and demos his olive oil pie-dough technique. It's pretty amazing to see how it's possible to use oil—a liquid!—and still get those pockets of fat that are necessary for flakiness. But I'm sure I couldn't duplicate it in my own kitchen without years of practice. We get an object lesson in underbaked pies when Chef assigns Katherine to keep an eye on the demo crust as it bakes. She pulls it from the oven as it begins to take on the color of a manila folder. When he sees it, he scoffs, tears it in two, and puts half back in the oven. When the second half is good and browned we do a compare and contrast. The underbaked crust is leathery and dry. It reminds me of some awful overworked cornmeal crackers I made once. The well-done crust is nutty, flaky, not at all overwhelmingly olive oil flavored. It would make fantastic crackers. In spite of the fact that we ate lunch just over an hour ago, no one can stop eating it.

⁂

P.M.

THIS AFTERNOON'S LUXURY activity is a dessert-wine tasting. It's run by a totally stereotypical British wine snob who talks about beneficial molds, hills next to bodies of water, and flavors of raisin, apricot, and green apple. There are a lot of pretentious comments from Maureen, who at dinner has shown herself to be the resident wine aficionada, and boneheaded questions from Derrick ("What's the name of that grape in other languages?"). My underdeveloped palate can't taste the fine distinctions—some wines are light and some are heavy, that's pretty much it for me. But I manage to make some of my own pretentious notes anyway: "apricots," "wet wool," "honey and apples, almost caramelized." Tee hee.

Dinner at American Bounty. They're not kidding about the bounty. Thank god the first course is a salad. A "steakhouse chopped salad," to be specific, which actually has iceberg lettuce in it. I am shocked—not because I disdain iceberg but because I thought the CIA would, for sure. But it's light and crunchy in that iceberg lettuce way, which everyone seems to be craving. (There are appallingly few vegetables on the menu here, and I think we're all feelin' the lack.) Then it's a Cornish hen on an incredibly rich bed of something made with corn and a hefty dose of cream. Dessert is a mixed berry cobbler with ice cream, a serving big enough for four. Over the twenty minutes we sit and talk, I end up cleaning my plate. I go back to my room and have a liver attack.

THURSDAY

A.M.

IT'S THE FIRST of two days of yeasted doughs, and I can barely contain my excitement. I've been reading about bread for months. This is really why I'm here. The class has been sneaking up on bread all week, asking off-topic questions about crustiness and open structure. Chef Henry tells us about his attempts to duplicate a steam-injected oven at home. All techniques have been unsatisfying thus far, so he intends to cut a hole in his oven through which he can stick the milk-steaming attachment from his cappuccino machine. I fear that if it works I'll want to try it too.

Down in the bakeshop, Derrick and I are assigned challah, which my esteemed partner insists on pronouncing as if its first syllable were the same as that in "cha-cha." Even though I keep saying it back to him in my own more authentic (though admittedly not properly throaty) pronunciation ("Have you ever made cha-la before?" "No, I've never made ha-la, but I have eaten a lot of ha-la."), he can't or won't pick up on it. Or maybe he just thinks he's right.

I share my pain with Maureen, who has been working next to me and Derrick all week and has noticed his preference for jawing with Chef over, say, helping me keep our station clean. (I believe my exact words were "If my idiot partner says 'cha-la' one more time, someone's going to die and I hope it won't be me.") She promises to take care of it, and lo and behold, during Chef's demo on how to do the traditional six-stranded braid, she pipes up. "Chef, what's the proper way to pronounce the name of this bread?" she asks earnestly, which makes me see immediately why she must be so good at keeping her clients happy at work.

Derrick lumbers about, *slooooooooowly* assembling our dry ingredients while I separate two dozen eggs to get the pint of yolks we need. We get it all together into the mixer and are mixing away when we notice quite a contrast with Lily and Fred's challah dough in the mixer next to us. Ours is wet and sticky, theirs is firm, firm, firm. We call Chef over. Looks like neither is really quite right, so he dumps all of the dough together to finish mixing. He tells us the texture differences could have been caused by a slight mismeasurement on both our parts, as little as a quarter-ounce of liquid in each case. For a formula that makes six pounds of dough, the thought that a variation of less than half an ounce of liquid could cause such drastic differences is both astounding and daunting.

P.M.

THE DOUGH ROSE over lunch (I had curried goat—richly fatty and surprisingly ungamey), and now it's time to shape it. Turns out I am laughable at the six-stranded braid, so much so that the chef observes, "Come on, you're supposed to be genetically predisposed to do this." I seek help from Jenn, who of course has turned out an impeccably braided loaf on the first try. Mine still ends up misshapen, but not shamefully so. (A week later, when I make challah back at my parents' apartment to be served at my nephew's bris, I just stick with a simple three-stranded braid and the loaves still look quite beautiful.)

We mix up the sponge for tomorrow's bread, which for me and Derrick is a semolina pizza/focaccia dough, and everyone makes a pie filling of his or her choice so that we can each bake a pie to take home tomorrow, using dough that's been chilling since it was made on Tuesday. *Mmmm, sour cherries.*

FRIDAY

A.M.

NO LECTURE TODAY. It's a production frenzy as we all finish our lean doughs (semolina for some, durum sourdough for others, and the pizza for us because Derrick was asking the chef about it all week like a man obsessed) and get them bulk-fermenting, then get to work shaping soft rolls and brioches and Danish and panettones and croissants. Chef Henry demonstrates about a kajillion techniques in the space of twenty minutes, then says, "Go! Let's get this all done!"

Much to my surprise, I find I'm adept at shaping the classic *brioche à tête*: Take a ball o' dough and make a dent at the one-third mark. Shmush with the side of your hand until you have something that looks like two different-sized balls connected by a small cord of dough. Press the smaller ball into the larger, making an indentation in the big one so there's a place for the small one to sit without being too squashed. Voilà. It's a lot more forgiving than the Danish, which I simply cannot form properly.

I have another crucial light-bulb-over-the-head moment concerning pie: It's not rolling that's my problem; it's the inferiority of my dough that's been the cause of my woes all along. No point in going to lunch today. We've got little pizzas going, plus bread, pastries, and the rest of the cookies that didn't get baked earlier in the week. *Mmm.* I realize I have never tasted an all-butter croissant before. Most in this country are made with at least some hydrogenated vegetable oil; it's cheaper and easier to handle. I suddenly understand what all the fuss is about.

P.M.

IT'S AN EMBARRASSMENT of baked goods, with several dozen loaves of sourdough, beautifully decorated with the spiral pattern from the bannetons they proofed in; eleven pies, including a monster deep-dish apple belonging to George (he must have brought his own pie tin, 'cause I've never seen anything like it); soft rolls in various knots and cloverleaf shapes; panettones of various sizes suspended upside down from skewers to cool; and, of course, countless plain, almond, and chocolate croissants, Danish of various flavors, and teeny brioches. In addition to the fresh-baked stuff, there are scones and biscuits and quick breads that were frozen on Monday and Tuesday. We're busy, gluttonous little beavers packing it all up to take home.

I ride to the train station with Lily and Fred, my bag overstuffed with three bakery boxes of Danish, cookies, scones, and biscuits; my cherry pie, which I hope I packaged well enough to keep the inevitable leakage off my clothes; a loaf of durum sourdough; and a plastic bag full of soft rolls and brioches. The thought of eating any of it is none too appealing—for once, I've had my fill—but I can't wait to get back in the kitchen and make more.

lessons from gabon

{ TEREZ ROSE }

I'LL NEVER MAKE fun of your meatloaf again, Mom. Just get me back to sample some. Five days into my two-year Peace Corps assignment in Gabon, Central Africa, I was ready to go home. Baked chicken, buttery garlic bread, green bean casserole, mashed potatoes and gravy . . . The thought of all I'd taken for granted plunged my diarrhea-ravaged stomach into further misery, as I stared at my plate of rice and mystery meat drowning in fiery sauce. *I would even settle for your Friday night fish sticks and tater tots, Mom.*

I grew up in the Midwest at the tail end of the Boomer era, under the motherly influence of Mrs. Paul, Mrs. Smith, Ore-Ida, and the Swansons. They were like family, benevolent aunts always there to assist my mother in her endless, nightly role of feeding eight children. She was old-school, staying at home to raise her oversized brood, but without nearby extended family to help. My father was not unsympathetic to her plight. Instead of building a mother-in-law unit, he built a freezer room to house my mother's greatest support system.

My mother had no time to peruse creative recipes or experiment in the kitchen. There were always dishes to wash, noses to wipe, fingerprint smudges to clean, arguments to break up, crying kids to hug. Every frozen or canned shortcut found a place in her kitchen. A meal of tater tots, broccoli, fish sticks, and cling peaches in syrup could be on the table in twenty minutes, leaving more time to fold laundry, vacuum, and herd little ones to bed. And yet, she managed to incorporate a few old-fashioned meals into our weekly repertoire, like Sunday roasts with onions in the gravy; thick, meaty spaghetti sauce with fragrant garlic bread on the side; casseroles that bubbled with cream and tangy cheese—never mind that the vegetables on the side were always canned or frozen and we had sandwich cookies for dessert.

I didn't think twice about leaving it all behind to join the Peace Corps in 1985. What twenty-two-year-old does? I was ready for a grand adventure, far beyond the confines of family and Kansas.

⁂

I LEARNED AFRICA'S first lesson quickly: eat to live, instead of live to eat. Food here was a necessity—not an indulgence, or a source of guilty pleasure. Gabon's main staples were rice and manioc, an indigenous tuber that is boiled, pounded, boiled again, pummeled, kneaded, then rolled into a banana leaf to form a baton of pale, stiff, nearly tasteless goop, visually reminiscent of the translucent pink erasers used by grade-school kids. One of these starches, accompanied by an ubiquitous, spicy tomato sauce, usually with some form of protein bobbing about (smoked fish, monkey, river rat in the village; beef, chicken, or fish in the cities), is what the average Gabonese eats. During my three-month training, it is what I ate too.

Culture shock and fear of the unknown produced a sick weepiness in me that made me want to stuff creamy casseroles into my body, wolf down burgers and fries, meals all unavailable here. To not have access to familiar foods was one of the worst feelings I'd experienced in my easy life. Food, I realized, had been my most loyal friend. It had sustained me through breakups and periods of angst, depression, boredom. It was something I could control and manipulate. Salt. Fat. Cheese. My pulse would quicken at the thought of the next meal. In Gabon, I didn't know what the next challenge would be or how I'd solve it. Now, when I needed comfort more than ever, my old friend had fled—to be replaced by monkey and manioc.

⁘

AFTER THREE MONTHS of Peace Corps training I received my teaching post, along with my own house. Amid continued homesickness, preparing my own food helped connect me once again to family, to control. In the kitchen that first night, I made canned corned beef and onions over rice. By normal culinary standards it was pretty forgettable, but the familiarity, the warmth of the food, comforted my heart as well as my stomach. It was canned. It was processed and salty, not spicy. It could have come from Mom's kitchen.

In Makokou, a provincial town of 6,000 surrounded on all sides by emerald rainforest, I struggled to acclimate. I still relentlessly craved the honest, predictable comfort of Mom's cream of mushroom soup–based creations (cream of mushroom soup being the key ingredient in any self-respecting midwestern cook's arsenal). As I ate corned beef and rice, bland fish and rice, spaghetti and rice, I dreamed of tuna noodle casserole, scalloped potatoes, green bean casserole with canned french-fried onions on top. In one sense, I was fortunate—I had an oven in my galley-sized kitchen, and a few battered pans. But there could be no casserole without Campbell's, which the local store shelves conspicuously lacked. *Baked chicken, then*, I thought. Another roadblock—in the provinces, chicken was hard to find and expensive. I found turkey wings, however, which I promptly baked Mom-style, dipped in flour and spices and basted with butter. When the familiar garlicky, rich smell of cooking poultry began to permeate the house, I almost wept with relief and nostalgia.

Although I loved my mother dearly, we never had that much in common. Her quiet, compliant nature paled against my flamboyant theatrics. Always warm and loving, she was emotionally elusive. She never confided in us and I never once saw her cry. Was this a result of her upbringing? A generational difference? Or did thirty years of raising nine kids, burying one as an infant, simply beat any subversive emotion out of her? The older I got, the more I wanted to know. In the years before I left I pestered her over dinner preparation. Did it make her nostalgic to prepare Swiss steak, one of the few recipes from her mother's kitchen? What were her childhood dinners like?

"Does the thought of cooking these same meals, day after day, ever make you want to freak out?" I tried once. "Don't you want to kick up your heels occasionally and try something wild and new?"

" . . . Honey, I don't know," she'd say with a puzzled smile. And that's all I got. How frustrating her responses were to someone like me, relentless until satisfied.

It was interesting to recognize that that's how I approached food too. I've always hungered to know why foods as basic as sugar cookies can vary so much by rendition, why some hollandaise sauces taste bland and heavy, while others are so exquisite, ethereal, and buttery. What was the secret of good food? With time on my hands in Gabon, I pored over the Betty Crocker cookbook Mom sent me. I tried new recipes, attempted dishes Mom had never made. Quiche. Fritters. Paella. Chicken tetrazzini. Sometimes I'd leaf through the cookbook and peruse recipes I didn't have the ingredients for: Oriental Veal Casserole (a rather frightening concept, incomprehensibly requiring cream of mushroom soup). Shrimp Rémoulade. Nesselrode Pie. (To this day, I don't have a clue what or who or where "Nesselrode" is.) Pumpkin Pie. On this last one, homesickness in November provided a powerful motivator to find substitutes for absent ingredients. I plucked a green papaya from a tree in my yard. Boiling and mashing it, I mixed it with evaporated milk, egg, sugar and spices. Trial and error finally produced the best pumpkin pie substitute in Central Africa. Mrs. Smith would have begged for the recipe.

During meals with friends featuring African food, I spent long moments in meditative silence, trying to define the flavors, to discern what made them so different from the foods I'd eaten growing up. The answer: peanut butter and lots of oil. Also *piment*, a chili pepper similar in heat to a habanero that lifted the blandness of rice and tomato sauce. The flavors that had evoked uneasiness upon my arrival now began to intrigue me.

·❖·

I ENCOUNTERED MANY roadblocks to my experiments, which pretty much defines life in Africa. The thermostat in my oven was broken. There were no frozen amenities in the local store, only lumpy, ice-crusted packages I learned to identify as turkey wings and on a good week, beef chunks or an occasional whole chicken. I had to make rice the old-fashioned way. It shocked me to discover how long it took, after the convenience of Minute Rice. It tasted better too, once it stopped sticking to the pan. Bit by bit, I modified American recipes with what was available and learned through experience how to gauge my oven temperature: I'd stick my head close, letting my face get the full blast of the heat. A 400° Fahrenheit oven blasts the face in a quick wave, so that the hair escaped from a ponytail waves back in retreat. A 375° oven is softer, more like an ocean swell. 450° is like a slap. Any higher, the eyebrows singe.

Spending time in the kitchen connected me to Mom. I saw more clearly how her personality manifested itself in her plain but comforting food, honestly and lovingly prepared. She found help where she could, quietly bearing the burden of cooking for a big family every night for over thirty-five years. I imagine her mother did the same. As I experimented in the kitchen, a benevolent spirit filled the air, the ghosts of my matrilineal ancestry, generations of women who have all used the available food to create a sense of home and family, compromising when need be. My mother left security and extended family behind when she moved 500 miles with her husband and six (soon to be seven) children. Her grandmother was torn from her German homeland. I'm certain she struggled with the unavailability of familiar kitchen staples just as I did in Gabon. We all learned to adapt and thrive.

The first year was the hardest. I wrote Mom asking for suggestions and she sent me some of her powdered shortcuts: Dream Whip instant whipping cream, Lipton Onion Soup mix, ground spices, dried cheese sauce. She mailed little packets of French's yellow mustard with a note about how the crew at the local McDonald's probably called her "that crazy lady who always asks for one hamburger and eight packets of mustard." I'd never heard her crack a joke or confide before—she was a different person on paper.

And then she sent the egg casserole recipe, the only casserole in her repertoire that didn't require cream of mushroom soup. In my hometown neighborhood, egg casserole was synonymous with celebration. Someone always brought it to brunches, to go with the muffins, Bloody Marys, and Screwdrivers. The dish was rich, oily, tangy, and substantial, with loads of cheddar cheese and pork sausage. My mother always made it for holiday breakfasts.

When I received the recipe, my heart leapt as I gazed at the index card with Mom's careful, familiar handwriting. *Home,* it whispered. I'd brought cheese from the capital city of Libreville, but in regards to the pork sausage, modifications were once again necessary. I fried canned corned beef (it was either that or turkey wings) in a pan with plenty of oil until the gooey rose-colored mush separated a bit and grew crispy. In place of Tabasco, I used *piment,* so hot one needs to chop it with protected hands (recognize the voice of experience speaking here). Having combined the fiery bits with oil, I now added a few drops to the meat. I mixed in eggs, milk, cheese, mustard, and bread, refrigerated it overnight and popped it in the oven on Sunday morning. The rich, buttery smell coming from the oven an hour later invaded my senses like a drug.

When I sat down and tasted the concoction, the flavors leapt out at me. I shut my eyes and let the cheesy richness transport me home: to the oversized dining table that sat twelve; to the adjacent gold and green print drapes that didn't quite match the industrial carpet beneath; to Mom, Dad, my seven siblings, and their kids in highchairs who banged spoons on trays, all raising their voices in order to be heard over the cheerful din. I opened my eyes to find Africa, where unknown trials awaited me. Parasites and insects were sure to compromise my health. Who knew if I'd make good friends in Makokou. But at that moment, I had my egg casserole. I took another bite and smiled.

⁜

SOMEWHERE DURING MY second year in Gabon, I went from simply accepting my culinary compromises to enjoying them. Like the locals, I regularly doused the plain food I made with *piment,* savoring the burn that made my eyes water and nose run. I learned to prepare fresh fish and other can-less meals. I snatched up avocados, mangos, guavas, and passion fruit—items I'd never used or even seen at home—whenever they appeared at the local market. On a daily basis I visited the local *boulangerie,* which produced surprisingly excellent baguettes.

Libreville, the capital city, hosted thousands of French expatriates. The French firmly embraced the "live to eat" philosophy, and no hardship post in Central Africa was going to keep them from living it. Stores catered to their tastes, providing olives; *pâté de foie gras;* tiny, tart *cornichons*—all new to my Midwestern palate. The cheeses alone were an education. (Back home, cheese meant Velveeta. My mom used to wave a cheese cutter through the orange loaf. She called her creation "nervous cheese," because of the squiggle shape, and served it as a side dish.) In Libreville, I discovered grating cheeses, semisoft cheeses, baking cheeses, unbelievably foul-smelling cheeses. Like all Volunteers, I learned to stock up on cheese, chocolate, and other French goodies whenever I visited.

Africa's more relaxed pace, combined with the French eating philosophy, produced long, lazy dinners with friends. Lingering over wine after plates were cleared, we argued about reincarnation, what made a good croissant, Western policy on developing nations, and why Regab, the Gabonese national beer, kicked Budweiser's ass. Candles, a necessary preventative measure for the frequent power outages, lit the animated faces around the table. As I brought out Pont-l'Évêque cheese and sliced mangoes for dessert, a voice whispered, "You don't need to long for home anymore. You *are* home."

⁂

AND THEN IT was time to leave my new life behind and return to Kansas. I wasn't prepared for the reverse culture shock. Without the *piment* I'd gotten used to, midwestern food seemed staid and lifeless. Mom's spaghetti sauce wasn't as satisfying, maybe because I'd learned that aged Parmigiano-Reggiano cheese worked better on top than Borden's grated domestic Parmesan *("New and improved, longer shelf life!"*). I was back to Minute Rice, frozen vegetables, tater tots, and fish sticks. Popping biscuits out of a can seemed absurd, almost surreal. My two-year absence had shown me, with painful clarity, mainstream Midwestern America of the '70s (Mom never really graduated to the '80s).

I tried to introduce the "new me" to the family. One night I made paella, accompanied by garden-fresh greens and avocados tossed with homemade vinaigrette. I'd procured crispy French baguettes. I lit candles. My dad tried to leave the table after shoveling down a plateful. I told him he had to stay for dessert. We needed to linger, drink coffee, and argue philosophy.

"Cheese for dessert?" my father spluttered when I brought Brie and grapes to the table.

"It's not orange," my sister complained. I grabbed a bag of Hershey's Kisses Mom kept around and bribed everyone to stay fifteen minutes longer. At our midwestern table, that was the best I would get.

Kansas betrayed me—or did I betray Kansas? Regardless, I had one consolation prize: My relationship with my mother had improved, now that we had cooking in common. She was happy to relinquish partial control of the kitchen as I continued to prepare side dishes more in line with my new tastes. As we puttered in the kitchen, she listened with rapt attention to my Africa stories, especially the ones detailing my kitchen disasters. (Dropping a full pot of spaghetti on the floor, seconds before serving it to a group, and serving it anyway; running out of propane for the oven midway through dinner party preparation; setting bread on fire, to name but a few.) Mom alone never tired of hearing them. My trick of successfully guessing the oven's temperature using my face endlessly entertained her. She loyally ate seconds when I made the family my African-style egg casserole, with corned beef and lots of Tabasco. (Corned beef, it turns out, is a poor substitute for pork sausage.) I'm sure my passionate nature baffled her, but I saw her girlish appreciation of the way I still insisted on candles at dinner and made Dad stay at the table longer. She wouldn't have done it on her own.

I tried once to branch away from our safe culinary conversations to ask her again if her never-ending job in the kitchen stifled a more creative, idealistic side of her. She gave me the same puzzled smile she always had and said, "Honey, I just don't think that way." I suppose that's one step up from saying, "Honey, I don't know." It eventually sank in. She wasn't introspective—in her era, that could be a dangerous thing. And I was—and could afford to be. We would always be two different people from two different generations.

⁘

IT'S BEEN FIFTEEN years since my return from Africa and twelve years since my mother died in her sleep, slipping away as uncomplainingly as she lived her life. I have few souvenirs of her—she wasn't a woman who believed in material possessions, sentimental knickknacks. For that reason, the egg casserole recipe card stands as one of my most precious mementos. Stained, dog-eared, and yellowing with age, Mom's elegant handwriting gracing the card, the recipe evokes memories of my youth, my struggles to adapt in a foreign place. It also represents the only casserole that made it into my adult repertoire, surviving the purge of my Midwestern palate.

Like the French, I still live to eat, celebrating life through food. However, I don't prepare what my mother and her generation produced. Early on, I sent Mrs. Paul, Mrs. Smith, and Ore-Ida packing. Tater tots, I told myself, along with canned biscuits and frozen broccoli, would never appear on my table. I've got many like-minded friends here in Northern California and we laugh together about surviving childhoods full of cream of mushroom soup and frozen atrocities. But surely my mother is up there laughing now as my son rejects my organic, seasonal creations in favor of what really interests him: frozen food. Chicken nuggets, hot dogs, frozen pizza—that's all he wants. Ore-Ida and the gang now get visitation rights. Once again, I yield, I compromise, and it makes life easier. *"Now you're getting it,"* Mom tells me.

mom's egg casserole

1 lb. bulk pork sausage, diced, browned and drained

6 slices white sandwich bread, cut into squares (no crusts)

2 cups milk

4 eggs, beaten

dash of Tabasco

1 tsp. dry mustard

1 tsp. salt

¼ lb. grated Velveeta or cheddar cheese

Mix all ingredients, pour into 8×8 pan and refrigerate overnight or twelve hours. Cover with foil. Bake at 325° for one hour. Remove foil for the last fifteen minutes. Casserole is done when center has set. Cool slightly and enjoy.

terez's african egg casserole

1 can corned beef

½ tsp. piment-oil mixture

2 T. peanut or palm oil

1 baguette, preferably not too stale

2 cups water

6 T. powdered milk

4 eggs, beaten

2 packets McDonald's prepared yellow mustard

1 tsp. salt

1 Bonbel cheese (in the red wax rind), chopped

Fry corned beef in oil (palm oil will have a stronger taste, but if it's all you have, it's all you have) until mixture becomes less gooey and crispy around edges. Break up into small pieces. When it vaguely resembles pork sausage, remove from heat and drain. Mix water with powdered milk, whisking out lumps. Take baguette and pluck out all the fluffy white stuff, leaving crust behind. (Save crust to slather with peanut butter for next meal.) Mix all ingredients and pour into any pan available (just make it work). Refrigerate overnight (assuming you have a refrigerator).

Next day, preheat oven, testing by holding face over open door. If heat blasts and is intensely uncomfortable, turn it down. If it's slow to hit face and feels more like a hot New York sidewalk in August, turn it up. Stick cookie sheet on top of pan for the first forty-five minutes (since no aluminum foil is available in the entire town). When incredibly good smell, reminiscent of home, wafts out of kitchen, check casserole. If burnt, too bad, live with it. If only half-cooked because your propane tank ran out midway and the town's general store is out of propane until next week, too bad, live with it. If it's cooked and doesn't jiggle in the middle, congratulate yourself and remove from oven. Cool slightly, if you have the patience, and enjoy.

cooking class

{ MICHELLE TEA }

I.

Dennis is my father and Louisa my mother. Louisa's name I've changed, because she is a good woman and horrified that I sit down in bars and coffeehouses, scrawling out the history of this family. Dennis remains himself, a darkly Polish man, mustached, always eating weird gross foods that he'd hoard, keep all to himself as if anyone in the family would want to take a bite. Tripe, for starters. What is it? I think it is intestines, but when I was little it was blubber, whale blubber, which I'd read about in school. How natives used it for candles and cooking grease. It seemed that my father liked to eat it. Long, bubbled strips of it quivered on the kitchen counter. I think he boiled it. It trembled, it was alive, like the Blob. It made sense that my father ate disgusting and mysterious things, because you are what you eat, I'd learned that, too, and my father was a mystery, one you didn't exactly want to figure out. Let him stay in the kitchen on a bright weekend, his day off, preparing his special foods with a can of beer gleaming beside him. Kielbasa was a Polish food, and that was only for him, too. Like a hot dog, but the skin was so hard you had to pop it with your teeth, which was frightening. It was like you had to kill it a bit to eat it. You knew that the food Dennis ate used to be alive, used to be an animal. It really seemed like dead stuff, unlike hamburgers, which just seemed like hamburgers, not dead cows. Sometimes Dennis's food *was* still alive when he brought it in the door. The snapping crabs and lobsters that lived for a bit in the bathtub, attempting to scramble up the porcelain slope, then skidding back into the basin. Thick rubber bands binding the lobsters' claws. It was like the zoo had come into our home, or the zoomobile—like the bookmobile but with small, strange animals instead of books. It had parked at my school once, and one by one classes were allowed to leave the building and climb on board to view tarantulas and lizards basking beneath heat lamps in little aquariums.

Dennis brought live animals home, into this house where there were no pets. A parakeet, for a minute, but it was loud and screechy, and would jump into its dish of seeds and run in place, scattering the tiny grains all over the place. The parakeet wanted out. It would stick its hooked beak through the bars and bite your finger. A ferocious little bird, lemon-limey, we got rid of it. Now these hard-shelled things clambered about in our bathtub. The scuttling crabs and the lumbering lobster. They'd go into the pot. When water began to boil and bubble, Dennis, like a witch, would drop them into the stew, and they would die there before us. We'd watch, me and Madeline, having been called into the kitchen to see it. I thought of Bugs Bunny in a roiling tub, carrots bobbing in the water like bath toys, how he'd outwit Elmer Fudd and be free again, not dinner. But the sea animals, we watched their shells redden and their eyes grow dull and smoked. They'd be dead then, almost ready to be eaten. Once, it was a lobster, still alive, its stiff tentacles whipping above the water like the limbs of a drowning man, and Dennis took the pair of metal tongs, the ones used to lift sweet ears of boiled corn from the pot, and he dipped the pinching tips into the blue gas flame and heated them, then clamped them on the lobster's twitching antennae. *That's the most sensitive part of the lobster,* he explained, enjoying this last, extra bit of pain before the creature expired. Later, he'd split their shells with a crack and tug out the puffy, white insides. He gutted the entire body—even the clattering claws were smashed open with the metal nutcrackers we used during holidays. He removed a long, slender bit of meat that had fit the shell of the claw exactly. It was like pulling fingers from a glove. Dennis mashed it up with mayonnaise and kept it in a Tupperware bowl in the fridge. He ate it on soft slices of Wonder Bread. It was for him and him alone. Dad food.

Dennis was Polish but from where in Poland I have no idea. His parents, my grandparents, were creepy, Old World novelties. They were the oldest of the old and I was scared of them, saw them only in rare photos. Dennis hated them. It was an alcoholic family, they all mostly hated each other. Dennis had a host of brothers— some I never met, some I saw sporadically. When Dennis was drenched with booze he'd get nostalgic and plan for a reunion. Then there'd be some new Polish men, all alcoholic, all rotting away slowly from various alcohol-related diseases: cirrhosis, diabetes. My family called it "Sugar." Lots of divorces in these men's lives, children who refused to talk to them. Eventually Dennis wouldn't want to either, and the men would vanish again.

Dennis would take us shopping, me and Madeline, to the special shops that sold his oddball snacks. Stop & Shop was good enough for normal stuff, but Dennis's strange palate required trips to butcher shops, where the hacked-up animals were splayed on ice: schools of dead-eyed fish, watery chunks of red, red meat, some with rocks of bone jutting out from them. The floors were wet and slippery, the air cold and heavy with a bloody smell you could taste, clammy on your lips. Dad's blubber would be laid out, too, like ribbons for a ghastly princess. A tank jammed with angry-looking crabs and lobsters, crawling around on each other. He'd point out his choices to the butcher, who would lift them, dripping, antennae flailing, and package them up. It was so weird to be back in the car with them, the shifting, moving packages. Live food. He'd take us into Martinetti's, where only bottles were sold. Row after row, and many enchanting—the glass extravagantly long at the neck, corked with wax, the labels old-looking, European. Dennis went to the back, to the refrigerated part, hauled a couple of six packs from the frost, and we were on to the next stop. Tripe, kielbasa, shellfish and beer.

II.

MEG WAS A big woman who was just fantastic-looking: robust, gold curls on her head fat as a baby's fist, twirling and bobbing like toys. Meg looked simply healthy in her body, despite the fact that she was, by neighborhood standards, fat. Bigger than my mother, who had taken to attending the twelve-step meetings at Overeaters Anonymous, adopting an OA-prescribed diet of chicken cutlet with raspberry vinaigrette dressing that was so exotic in its simplicity, infinitely preferable to the greasy meat combinations prepared separately for the rest of the family. A regular box-and-can dinner for me and Will and Madeline, the kids, and then this clean-looking, pink-drizzled delicacy for herself. It sat on her plate like a food photo from a women's magazine, elegant and sparse. Occasionally I would nibble at her sweet and tangy meat. *Get away,* she'd swarm in like a mama animal protecting sustenance. *This is MY food.* Sometimes Ma would rear up against the ritual of sharing that motherhood had forced her into. Nothing my mother possessed was hers alone. I'd rummage through her dresser for sweaters, for underwear in desperate times. I'd swipe her fantasies from the dirty books she hid, and steal cigarettes from her pack when she locked herself in the bathroom to pee—I took everything. Sometimes she'd rebel, like with her sweaters. She hated having to charge into my room and pull through the lumps of clothes and junk on the floor, looking for what was hers. *This is MINE,* she'd lay a thick boundary of words in the home, a tiny verbal fence that would keep us, for a moment, out of her bedroom, away from the refreshing new clothing options stuffed in her drawers. It was like the tits we never got to nurse in the hospital became all she owned—everything she had was ours, and she didn't have much, but occasionally I would want it. Like the citrusy chicken that tasted so good. She ate it proudly as we wiped grease from our chins with our wrists. Us, her three-headed offspring with the many grasping hands. She had so few opportunities to separate herself from our need, to not be a mom, and her entire non-mom identity became symbolically encapsulated in that one sweater I was not allowed to wear. The heavy knit one with colors that faded so gently from the collarbone's pink, to darling blue, to the hem's arresting purple. The perfect sweater. Or the chicken, trim and graceful in its gelatinous raspberry pool. It was for Ma and her body, which we had imposed upon for so long, our basic economic drag propelling her to supermarket aisles stocked with boxes of Hamburger Helper, the cheapest ground beef, tiny nodules of fat glistening out from the moist red squiggles.

III.

MY MOTHER REALLY liked that movie *Stella,* a 1990 remake of an old Barbara Stanwyck movie, with Bette Midler in the starring role. Ma had a dramatic fear that she herself was a Stella figure, and that the tragedies of class betrayal would be sprung upon her by us, her daughters. We would marry into wealth; ashamed of our white-trash, Chelseaen upbringing we would disown her, Louisa, our mother. She would give us up in a final grand gesture of maternal self-sacrifice and self-loathing, she would peek through the church window as we moved without her into a life of riches. We would be in big white gowns, Cartier tiaras twinkling on twists of hair. Something like this would happen. Of course, my recent lesbianism threw a bit of a wrench into this ruinous fantasy, but Steph was loaded, and it showed. My mother didn't want to discuss her, though it was clear that a lot of questions rolled through her mind. Occasionally, one would tumble out: *Where is she from? Oh, Connecticut. What do her parents do?* Stuff like that. It was apparent to me that Ma was put off less by Steph's baseball hat with the word "Dyke" stitched onto the brim, than she was by Steph's wealthy background. When I'd brought her to the confessional table, Steph had sat in her wooden chair with a steely, detached look on her face, unspeaking. I read her visible arrogance as that of a Sapphic warrior forced to face another brutal example of how men ruin lives; to Ma it was the face of a rich girl sitting in a ramshackle kitchen, taking in the grease-stained curtains, the torn corners of linoleum tiles—a voyeur to the shameful struggles of a dysfunctional working-class family.

I was conflicted about Steph's being rich. Sometimes it made me feel grumpy and resentful, but I kept it to myself. Me and Steph bickered enough without my having issues about her wealth. Sometimes where she came from seemed irrelevant, meaningless, occasionally I thought it was interesting, like having a friend from Europe. In high school I'd hung out briefly with Tanya, who was from France, and I thought that was really exciting. I would introduce her to people, saying, This is Tanya, she's from France! I didn't understand why she wanted me to stop. I never introduced Steph by saying, This is Steph, she's rich! but I would refer to myself as "white trash," and Steph and her friends were bothered. *I don't like to hear you putting yourself down,* Brad said. But I hadn't been. It was like being Polish, or a Dyke. How could I have thought that a white-trash party would be fun? I had thrown one. At my mother's house, while she was out of town with Will, back when me and Steph had first started going out. I put deviled ham on Saltines, with little bits of olive. I cooked Tuna Helper on a pot on the stove. I put on my mother's clothes: stirrup pants and flat-heeled shoes, a thin gold chain with its clump of twinkling charms—"#1 Mom," an Italian horn even though we were Irish, a teddy bear. The guests were Steph and Dinah, Brad and his new boyfriend. They didn't get it, they were rich kids. I brought a plastic bowl of bright orange macaroni and cheese into the parlor, where everyone was watching the vice-presidential debate on TV. They were laughing at Perot's running mate, that senile old guy. None of us could get over him. This was slightly before our group plunge into vegetarianism, but Steph, Dinah and Brad wouldn't eat the food I brought out. They were laughing at everything. Laughing with, laughing at—I understood the difference, and it was unexpected. My mother's worn shoes were tight at my toenails, her weighted necklace swung out when I bent to place the food on the table. I was a monkey shelling peanuts. I was my mother, I was Stella Dallas. Brad's new boyfriend was from Idaho, he had just come out of the closet and was all big-eyed, blue-eyed and blond. Like all of Brad's boyfriends, he looked just like Brad. He was eagerly eating the Tuna Helper, and they were making faces and laughing at him. *You're not supposed to eat it! He doesn't get it!* He was like Perot's running mate.

I sat on the floor and ate some deviled ham off a cracker. If you could forget about how the stuff looked when you first opened the can, the translucent gel clumped to the sides of the can, if you could forget about that first part and stir it all in, then deviled ham could be quite tasty. Salty on the crackers with the pickled bit of olive. *Eeeew,* said Steph as she scrunched up her face, laughed. They all left shortly, to go dancing. I stayed behind in my mother's empty house, Steph wanted a night out with *her friends.* I was alone in a kitchen that stank of warm tuna. If Ma had seen me, there in her pumps, making a joke of her to my new friends. I walked into the bedroom that smelled of her smell, unclasped the necklace and placed it gingerly on her dark bureau. Before Brad left he had taken a bunch of pictures hanging in the hallway and turned them all upside down on the wall. Then he'd stolen one of my mother's figurines. She had tons of them—Precious Moments, ducks, bunnies. Sweet children, with bonnets and puppies. Brad put one in his pocket and left. He gave it back to me later. He just thought it'd be funny to steal one for a while.

sex on a platter

{ KATE CHYNOWETH }

THE FOODS OF romance—chocolate-dipped straw-berries, fresh oysters, caviar, chilled Champagne—seem so icono-graphic now that one wonders how it ever could have been otherwise. Yet, in Victorian England, glasses overflowed with mead, a fermented honey drink with spices and citrus, not dry French bubbly. Dessert brought transparent pudding, with almonds and raisins glistening through a clear jelly mold, not triple-chocolate orgasm cake or passion fruit crème brûlée. While culinary ideals change with the times, the notion that certain foods carry roman-tic panache does not. Today, the culture of amorous eats looms large over anniversaries, wedding days, and romantic dinners, as it has for centuries. Seduced by the idea that rare and expensive delica-cies encourage intimacy more than, say, sliced bread, celebratory couples indulge in tiny piles of sturgeon roe and other treats, com-pletely unabashed by the breathtaking prices. Leave the daily grind of your dinner table behind—so the logic goes—and unbridled romance will result.

Given this, it's easy to imagine how, for a freelance writer like me, landing a job updating a well-known romantic travel guide to the Northwest engendered visions of gourmet indulgence. After marking time for years with morning toast and evening pasta washed down with bargain red wine, my just desserts had arrived, literally, and would soon be sliding down my throat at fine restaurants and superlative B & Bs. The research seemed as simple as hitting the road with my fun-loving—albeit gastronomically conservative—boyfriend for some amorous culinary adventures. The timing was perfect: Lowell, who was going through a slow period in his chemistry PhD research, seemed eager to make a getaway.

The break from our eating routine promised an ardent thrill. I'd been watching Lowell eat Cheerios almost every morning for nearly five years, and openly condemned his lack of interest in breakfast alternatives. I delighted in the chance to deviate from our norm, and suppressed my worries that Lowell's regular habits might interfere with our romantic dining quest. I should have considered a lesson I learned while single: Finding romance, and searching for it, can be (and usually are) mutually exclusive.

Nonetheless, my hopes remained high as I started to plan romantic itineraries around my territory of Washington, Oregon, and British Columbia. The possibilities dazzled: five-star inns perched on cliff edges, cozy mountain retreats, luxury lodges accessible only by float plane, and bed-and-breakfasts run by Cordon Bleu–trained chefs. Everywhere the restaurants promised romance. For a girl who loves good eats as much as I do, it sounded heavenly.

One Saturday morning, Lowell peered over my shoulder as I typed out the itinerary for our ten-day trip to British Columbia's remote Gulf Islands. He raked one hand through his uncombed sandy hair and blinked his blue eyes hard, as if trying to solve an equation.

"Is our every meal for ten days really *scheduled?*"

"Of course not," I lied. "We'll have lots of free time."

⁙

AS I CONTINUED my research, an unwelcome truth was becoming as clear as if my old junior-high Magic 8-Ball had spelled out the message: I was a rube about romance travel. I'd naively imagined that our idyllic dinners would be simple equations of wine and food enjoyed in excellent company. Alas, I'd neglected perhaps the most important goal: finding spots with kiss-worthy ambience.

Ah, ambience. The shadowy other half of any romantic meal. Important as, if not more important than, the food itself, ambience encompasses décor, lighting, artwork, music, flowers, and even service (how politely you are greeted and seated, how quickly the server drapes a napkin over your lap). The final, and most ephemeral, aspect of ambience is a combustible compound of tone, mood, and setting. For the romance researcher, then, the first order of business is finding waterfront views, blazing fireplaces, secluded tables for two, and red velvet drapes. In my efforts to hunt down ambience of the most sublime degree, I quickly discovered that, as oysters are standard romantic comestibles, formal dining rooms are standard romantic backdrops—as if the mere presence of a man in lapels could summon Cupid himself. In fact, I discovered, half the highly "romantic" restaurants on my Gulf Islands agenda require men to wear dinner jackets. (Lowell's idea of formal attire is a fleece jacket that hasn't pilled, yet he stayed relatively calm when I broke this news. His sole comment, "It's not really vacation if I have to dress up," struck me as a quiet rebellion that would, at some point during the trip, cause an unpleasant scene between us.)

I also became acquainted with a few other established clichés, including but not limited to the idea that, of all cuisines, formal French is the most romantic. And although I personally see little charm in eating strange animal parts like beef tongue or veal heart, then groaning my way through a cheese course while a stiff, tuxedoed waiter hovers over me, I dutifully kept these restaurants on my lists. Next, I grappled with the time-honored assertion that seven courses are more romantic than five; five more romantic than three; and three more romantic than one. While this prejudice toward stuffing oneself strikes me as less than sensible, given the aerobic aspect of certain romantic post-prandial activities, I had a job to do, and it wasn't to re-invent romance. Surely, with enough good humor, Lowell and I would have fun within the clichés, culinary overkill or not. I prepared myself for evenings of progressive eating.

Mornings of progressive eating were also on the schedule. Five-course breakfasts came with every single "romantic" overnight stay—and unfortunately, on some mornings, I'd been forced to schedule two breakfasts—one at our accommodation, and one elsewhere. While this now strikes me as insane, it sounded pleasant at the time. We would wake with coffee and scones, I'd thought, then meander to our next destination and enjoy a full breakfast around ten. In fact, I had no choice but to sign on for this schedule, as our limited time in the islands forced my hand. Breakfast was an ideal way to meet hosts and experience a place without having to spend an entire night, and doubling up was the only way to cover all the B & Bs on my list. I downplayed the tight eating itinerary to Lowell, ignored the stab of guilt, and prayed that copious amounts of juicy ham and crisp bacon would save the day.

Our first night in the Gulf Islands, we stayed on the grounds of a secluded vineyard that overlooked a valley where, around sunset, we actually spotted two bald eagles soaring among the dark green firs. In the morning, strong coffee magically arrived at our door along with the newspaper and a charming handwritten menu detailing our feast of local berries, hazelnut scones, and Northwest eggs Benedict. The food was sheer delight. A single, poached egg—perfectly cooked—laid on the thinnest slice of salmon lox, and topped with just a dash of light, steaming hot, lemony hollandaise. Our afternoon hike to a high, rocky bluff with views of B.C.'s northern snow-capped mountains replenished our appetites. We spent the evening at the local French bistro, charmed by its tiny waterfront dining room and spare, lovely food presentation: for me, an elegant pasta with thinly sliced truffles and Pecorino Romano; for him, a perfectly browned roasted rack of lamb. The experience wasn't entirely romantic, due to my incessant critique. *Wasn't that open kitchen unreasonably noisy? Did he believe, as I did, that the owner's untalented child had painted that terrible horse-farm mural on the wall? Why in the world couldn't they offer more than two wines by the glass?* By the time the slices of moist and luscious lemon cake arrived for dessert, my outbursts had subsided. Later, we would look back and consider the meal to be the most idyllic repast of the trip.

--:--

WE AWOKE THE next morning at 4 A.M. to Canadian radio blaring from the bedside alarm. Our dismay at the problematic early hour was only compounded by our dry mouths and throbbing heads, the predictable result of sharing a bottle of red wine and numerous snifters of cognac the previous evening. As Lowell put the bags into the trunk, and I rather frantically pawed through my overstuffed tote bag for the folder containing the day's schedule, our vineyard hostess appeared like a breakfast angel offering us a ribbon-tied bag filled with goodies. We unpacked the picnic in the ferry line, and, from our bucket seats in the car, watched dawn spill across the choppy, gray-blue Strait of Georgia. That our first destination on the next island was a five-star B & B—and a five-course breakfast—didn't prevent us from tearing into the apricot scones, homemade jam, Devonshire cream, chunks of ripe cantaloupe, and slices of rich, salty ham. We downed our coffee, and polished off every bite.

The ferry deposited us at the next island within the hour, but despite this timely arrival, we immediately ran behind schedule. Unable to locate the printed directions in my bag, I took the wrong turn out of the boat terminal, and immediately became lost on the island's unmarked dirt roads. As I reversed the car out of several dead ends in a row, cursing, I unbuttoned the straining waistline of my jeans.

"If I'm not hungry, you can't possibly be," Lowell said. He sat in the passenger seat with his eyes closed as if that might shut out the violence of my hapless driving.

I cracked my window for air.

"We don't have to eat. I just need to check this place out."

Finally, Lowell spotted signs for the B & B and we followed them until we turned off the washboard road and descended a smooth blacktop driveway. At its bottom, a massive house perched on an oceanfront cliff like a spaceship, all swooping modern lines and blinking windows. The woman who answered the door wore black leggings and a long teal sweater; her stiffly sprayed blonde hair parted in two smooth wings from the center of her forehead, and she wore my southern grandmother's shade of bright coral lipstick.

"Welcome, welcome." She ushered us in. "Now you two must be starving. Go ahead, have a seat!"

Lowell looked ready to run, so I took his hand firmly in mine. We followed her into the dining room.

"So glad you made it," she said, "I've been cooking all morning. Not many guests in the off-season. It's good to get back in the kitchen. What are you waiting for? Please, sit down."

We sat down as if we were about to hang in the gallows, rather than eat breakfast to Mozart with a spellbinding ocean view.

Heaping bowls of cranberry-cashew granola, broiled grapefruit, baskets of muffins, and ice cream sundae glasses filled with sliced fruit crouched by each of our place settings.

Lowell drank coffee while I started tearing one of the baseball-sized muffins into smaller pieces.

Before I had time to pretend further, the hostess put a plate in front of me. It was covered with a silver dome.

"Just to warn you," she said, "I'm the kind of cook who takes risks in the kitchen." She smiled. "This dish is creative, but it's always a big success. It's kind of like eggs Benedict, but with salmon. It's a Northwest twist—I invented it."

She pulled the dome off my plate with a flourish, and revealed airplane hangar–sized chunks of hot pink smoked salmon, topped with three eggs and drowned in buckets of hollandaise. I could just make out the limp English muffin, swimming below the surface.

I didn't dare look at Lowell's face when she unveiled his plate.

⁂

THAT NIGHT, WE dined in the restaurant of a new boutique hotel, a grand room encased in glass. Outside, the full moon laid down an avenue of light on the water, and ferries sailed by, trimmed with festive white lights. Lowell's mood was triumphant, since his refusal to wear a shirt and tie at my suggestion had been robustly justified by the Bermuda shirt–clad tourists at the surrounding tables. My fancy light wool trousers itched my legs.

For romantic research purposes, I felt compelled to order the oysters, although I couldn't actually touch them once they arrived, each nearly the size of a steak and glistening in grayish white liquor. I made a mental note to mention somewhere in my write-ups that huge Pacific oysters lack the romance of tiny, sweet Kumamotos. The arrival of my over-done slab of Pacific salmon did little to increase my appetite. However, I was pleased to see Lowell releasing some pent-up aggression in a knife-and-fork battle with his overcooked steak. We skipped dessert, and fled to our threadbare Victorian B & B. In the room, Lowell immediately went to the antique sideboard for the flask of amber sherry.

"Let's drown our sorrows," he said.

We clinked glasses, and each took a sip.

"I didn't know sherry could go bad," I said.

Lowell put down his glass carefully, then threw himself on the four-poster king-sized bed, and pronounced he couldn't wait to get home and live on peanut butter and pizza.

⁘

BY THE NEXT morning, I had developed a serious guilt complex about making my beloved partner suffer with me through this hellish food tour. It was only Day Four of our ten-day trip, and so far the food had been both awful and unduly plentiful (the vineyard breakfast and dinner at the French bistro were the sole exceptions). But there was no time for apologies: We were expected downstairs for breakfast in the dimly lit Victorian dining room.

Paul, our bearded host, gestured with quote marks in the air as he described the signature morning dish we were about to enjoy—an eggs Benedict "wrap"—a neat pink bundle of sundried tomato tortilla stuffed with scrambled eggs and smoked salmon, topped with a slump of hollandaise sauce that inexplicably resembled mustard both in consistency and color.

As covertly as possible, I split the tortilla down the middle, and extracted some pristine, sauceless eggs.

Paul said, "Don't you like hollandaise?"

His wife, Becky, cut in. "Of course she likes hollandaise," she gushed, "But, honey, us girls have to watch our figures." She looked at Lowell, who hadn't yet touched his plate. "See, now here's a tall guy. Count on him to finish everything."

He opened his mouth to protest.

"Don't worry," Becky said. "There's more in the kitchen."

⋯

THE FOLLOWING DAY, dawn found us in yet another ferry line—this time we were bound for the Gulf Islands' most remote outpost. We ignored all but the coffee in the ferry picnic packed by our hosts; after the rotten sherry and the viscous hollandaise, we felt less than confident about their gastronomic savvy. The usual reason to hold back was also at play: Our first order of business on the next island was breakfast at a rustic B & B far removed from the island's sole tiny town.

Upon arrival, I had the feeling that Barbara and Philip, our hosts, hadn't seen anyone but each other in quite a while. They seated us in a small, overheated dining room crammed with a large table set with linen and silver and a looming antique harp. Framed photographs of obscure German harpists took up the better part of the wall.

"It's my specialty to host harpists," Barbara said. "Before the accident, I owned horses. Now, it's all about harp music."

My boyfriend shot me a nervous look. The accident?

Philip, the husband, had disappeared to retrieve something in the kitchen, and now returned, pushing dramatically through the swinging doors, carrying a silver tray with two porcelain ramekins.

"Voila!" he said. "Sexy oatmeal!"

I searched for words and settled on, "How romantic."

"Smother anything with whipped cream and it's sexy, right?" Philip winked at his wife. "Or anyone."

Barbara said, "Oh, Phil, stop flirting."

My boyfriend looked dazed. I poured him some coffee from the insulated thermos. I nudged at my ramekin and the crown of whipped cream and strawberry sauce wobbled. I didn't see any sign of boiled oats.

Barbara said, "You two enjoy. We'll give you a chance to try this before we bring in our special pièce de résistance."

Which, as it turned out, was eggs Benedict with smoked salmon.

I had just finished choking half of it down, when somehow, trying to take off my sweater, I knocked the plate with my elbow. It crashed to the floor in a glory of broken china and egg yolk.

My boyfriend laughed.

I cursed. "It's not funny," I said.

He said, "Would it be wrong if I did that 'by mistake', too?"

I crouched down and started swabbing at the spreading mess with my napkin, trying to prevent the sauce from pooling around the intricately carved base of the prized harp. Nobody answered when I knocked on the swinging door into the kitchen, so I looked through the porthole window. The lovebirds were dancing a waltz. I knocked and then stuck my head in the door.

"I had an accident."

Philip said, "Ha, did you forget your diaper this morning?"

"Ha," I echoed flatly. "No, I dropped my plate."

"Philip," said Barbara, "don't make fun. I'll be right there with a cloth."

We both down got down on our knees and cleaned up the mess. Then she straightened, and said, "Okay, let's make you another breakfast."

"Please don't go to the trouble."

"Oh, it's so easy," she said. "We can just nuke some sauce and poach a couple eggs."

"No, really, that sounds like a hassle," I said, panicked, "I've had plenty to eat."

"It will be done in a jiffy. You just relax now, and have a muffin."

She disappeared again into the kitchen.

Lowell said, "That's right, have a muffin."

"You're finally enjoying yourself, aren't you."

"It's terrible to see you suffer." He smiled.

When my second breakfast arrived, I spooned half the serving into my napkin and slid the wet bundle into my purse. There would be other purses; one more taste of hollandaise sauce would be the end of my self-respect.

❖

THAT NIGHT, WE cancelled our fine dining reservations and went to the local burger joint instead. We sat in the warm dusk outside on an old wooden deck filled with a profusion of potted red geraniums, inhaled the scent of fried food and salt water, and watched the ferry boats cross the sparkling channel.

It was a sensible burger and beer for Lowell, but I ordered badly, and watched my plate of bland, gritty pesto linguine congeal as everyone else watched the sun sink in the west, and joyfully licked their fingers. The Merlot was corked. I ordered the beer I should have had to begin with.

I said, "Elusive quarry, the romantic meal."

"Maybe we should stop trying," he said.

"It's that simple," I said.

"Yes," he said. He had ketchup on the side of his mouth, and, for the first time in days, he looked happy.

# of cabbages and kings

{ THERESA LUST }

SAUERKRAUT IS NOT a dish you will find on too many American dinner tables these days. Frankly, it suffers from a frumpy image. Sauerkraut is something that waits limp and forgotten in a cafeteria buffet. Something Opal and Mavis dish up at the Grange for a Friday night supper. Definitely not something you'd serve on a first date. Impress your new sweetheart with a platter of thyme-roasted squab on a bed of couscous by all means, but do not set out a bowl of sauerkraut.

Sauerkraut is not epicurean fare upon which you dine, it is fodder upon which you subsist. Its origins date back to the Chinese, who fed cabbage preserved in wine to workers on the Great Wall. Sauerkraut migrated west in the baggage of the Tartar horsemen; they made it their sustenance when they invaded central Europe. Pliny mentions that the Romans ate cabbages preserved in oil and saltpeter during the winter months. And sauerkraut was partially responsible for Captain James Cook's triumphant second voyage around the world. He insisted it be included on his ship's list of provisions, and its high vitamin C content kept his men from coming down with scurvy.

The word "sauerkraut," which means "sour cabbage," comes from the Germans; the dish had become an integral part of their cuisine by the seventeenth century, as well as a peasant staple in Old World regions from Alsace to Estonia. Long northern winters kept the farmer from growing warm-weather crops like figs and artichokes, but his hearty cabbages could thrive in a short, cool growing season. When his wife preserved the cabbages in salt, she could count on the food in the larder to last the winter. And when the farmer's sons and daughters gathered their bags for America, they did not forget how they had feasted like kings and queens on humble cabbage.

When these immigrants arrived, Americans belittled them for their thick accents and tattered clothes, but they welcomed sauerkraut with open arms. The fare of slaves and paupers! It's a wonder they allowed it on their plates, but pile it on they did. Sauerkraut became a mainstay of the frontier. Housewives in South Dakota stored it in the root cellar, in between the crock of pickles and the sack of turnips. And in the city, sauerkraut became a staple of the neighborhood delicatessen. Proprietors in Brooklyn packed it between slices of corned beef and pumpernickel, or tucked it alongside mustard-slapped kielbasa cradled in a bun. Not even the War to End All Wars could snuff the American flame of passion for sauerkraut. The national dish of Germany? Not to worry. They changed its name to Liberty Cabbage and helped themselves to seconds.

This passion for sauerkraut proved to be no more than passing fancy. Food fashions, like hemlines, have always been subject to popular whim; they change at the drop of a kitchen knife. Liberty Cabbage has become passé. We may now eat *pad thai* and Jamaican jerked sausage, but sauerkraut is no longer in vogue.

This fact I understood all too clearly when I entered the cooking profession. I regarded my own fondness for sauerkraut as a sign of an uneducated palate. I felt it a handicap, indeed, to have been weaned on home cookin' instead of haute cuisine. Yet I managed to master the Mother Sauces in the kitchen with ease. I perfected the art of whisking while making sauce béarnaise. It's all in the wrist. I made a shallot and vinegar reduction over a high flame, and learned to spot the precise syrupy instant to swirl in the butter so as not to break my *beurre blanc*.

Since I knew I could not really learn to cook until I learned to taste, I took great pains to keep my palate in a rarefied culinary atmosphere. Instead of fried eggs at breakfast, I ate *quiche Lorraine*. No milk for me, I drank Perrier. A restaurant hamburger with French fries? How common. Bring me *entrecôte*, grilled rare, please, with a side of *pommes frites*.

But try as I might, I could not elevate my taste buds to the proper haute plane. The caviar that we oh-so-sparingly spooned atop poached fillet of salmon? To me, it was bait for a trout. And the crystal clear pheasant consommé with julienne carrot and leek? I preferred my mother's chicken soup.

It was a hard fact to accept. I did not inherit a silver palate through good breeding, and I could not create one through perseverance. I blame the whole sorry truth on my grandmother's garden.

That garden was not for cultivating a taste in caviar, it was for cultivating cabbages and beans. I look back on it and see dinner still growing in the soil. I understand her garden now as a connection to the land, a source of bounty and synchrony with the seasons. I'll confess that growing up, I didn't always see it that way. I can just about hear my exasperated mother saying, "Would you like me to call your Nana on the phone and tell her you won't eat the carrots she grew in her garden with her own sweat and tears? I didn't think so. Now you clean your plate." Or, at fourteen and miserable, how I wished my dopey mother would just buy her vegetables at the grocery store like everybody else's mom, and quit dragging me out to the farm to help with the weeding.

But after I left home and started cooking for myself, I realized the wealth of fresh flavors I had taken for granted in my grandmother's garden. That garden is why my preferences run toward tender young peas, shelled outdoors in June, eaten raw, two pods for the basket, one for me. It is why I relish the first red potatoes of the season, boiled until their jackets burst, then rolled in melted butter and fresh chopped parsley. And it's why I know how to savor a good, ripe tomato. Not a hothouse, not a hydroponic, but a fat beefsteak, plucked from the vine on an August afternoon, and eaten on the spot, with its sun-warmed juices dribbling down my chin.

And because that garden teemed with cabbages, I have a penchant for what some would call a paltry dish of sauerkraut. One bit conjures up vegetable gardens, 100-degree-in-the-shade afternoons, earthenware crocks, and warm soil under bare feet. It also summons up visions of my grandmother, who has put up quite a bit of sauerkraut in her day.

In the sprawling countryside of eastern Washington State where she grew up, making sauerkraut was just what farmwives did, usually after they canned tomatoes and right before they made applesauce. Her tattered loose-leaf notebook bulges with the recipes she has collected during a lifetime of preserving summer harvests. Page after page, she has jotted down recipes in her tidy, schoolgirl script. A few brittle sheets reveal her mother's hand in blotted India ink. Green Tomato Relish, Dilly Beans, Pickled Beets, Piccalilli, Pear Honey, Strawberry-Rhubarb Jam. She never will forgive herself for losing that old recipe for Muzzy's Brandied Fruit Compote. It went to the grave with her mother, rest her soul, and now it's gone for good.

One thing she's not sure she ever had is a recipe for sauerkraut.

Heaven knows, she might have a copy stashed around somewhere. No need for one, really. Sauerkraut has just two ingredients: fresh cabbage and salt.

Nana has the ingredients on her mind this late August morning. An entourage of relatives has assembled in her backyard— including my mother, my three sisters and me—and we are ready to make sauerkraut. I'm especially excited this year, because I'm eleven, and that's old enough to grate the cabbage. The cabbages wait in a wheelbarrow by the picnic table. Thirty tight, green heads, cut from the garden before breakfast, already warm from the sun. And it promises to be a hot one. Not yet ten o'clock, but yesterday's roses are dropping their petals, and the meadowlark is done singing at dusk.

A young cousin gives the pile a good sluice with the garden hose. He has been instructed by Nana not to go getting them too clean, though, for it's the good germs on the leaves that make for sauerkraut in the first place. So he soon turns the spray on his brother, who runs squealing across the lawn.

The benevolent germs in question are *Leuconostoc mesenteroides* and *Lactobacillus plantarum*. They have a predilection for saline solutions. A crock of salted cabbage is an immense prairie for them to homestead according to some molecular version of Manifest Destiny. The metabolic product of their toil is an enzyme called lactic acid, which ferments the cabbage and results in the characteristic taste and texture we've come to call sauerkraut.

Nana is no scientist, but she knows a good germ when she tastes it. One by one, we remove the loose outer leaves from each cabbage. With dishtowel, apron corner or shirttail, we wipe from the crisp heads any last traces of soil. We do not call it dirt. Dirt is what sticks underneath your fingernails or behind your ears. But when it plays host to the vegetables you've pulled from your garden, you call it soil.

One aunt halves the cabbages with brisk strokes of her kitchen cleaver, and another carves out the thick cores with a paring knife. Nana shreds the heads into slaw with the kraut-cutter that had been her mama's.

A kraut-cutter is a metal grating contraption. It is an arm's length long, and the span of an outstretched hand wide. Kraut-cutters are hard to come by these days, although you can pick one up at a flea market if you're lucky. Nana, who is now eighty-some, has told me I can have hers someday, but she's not finished with it just yet. Kraut-cutters are the instrument of choice when it comes to making sauerkraut, for they quickly turn the cabbage into shreds as thin as quarters, which encourages the osmotic flow of juices that starts the fermentation. A well-honed kitchen knife can do the job, but be careful to cut fine slices, or your cabbage won't juice-up, and it will mold instead of ferment.

We set to grating in Nana's yard. Mother after daughter after aunt after cousin, we spell one another, grating away until our respective old or young arms give out—Hold your hand away from the blade, dear, you'll slice your finger to the bone if you're not careful. Part orchestra, part assembly line, the resonant rap of cleaver on cutting board and the washboard rasp of cabbage against grater keep time.

My mother measures out slaw, five pounds to the batch, on an old grain scale. She dumps it into a metal washtub, throws in three tablespoons of pickling salt, and works it together with her hands, really roughs it up until clear juices stream forth and foam bubbles on the surface. Three or four pairs of young cousins' hands help out, squeezing the cabbage between stubby fingers, and packing it into a ten-gallon earthenware crock. They steal away handfuls of cool, crisp cabbage, dripping with brine. Gritty undissolved crystals stick to small fingers, then melt on warm tongues. A little one starts to cry, poor dear has a cut on her thumb. The salty brine stings deep and Nana says, Come now, honey, nothing a Band-Aid and a kiss won't mend.

Hard telling if some of us—the grandchildren—aren't more trouble underfoot than we are help. Which is perhaps why no one seems to mind when a few half-pints lose interest and bound off to the corn rows. The rest of us grate and pack, grate and pack, into the afternoon. It takes two aunts to haul the crock off to the cellar, then Nana presses a clean muslin cloth over the slaw, saturating it in the foamy brine. On top of the cloth she places a large plate, then fills a gallon Mason jar with water and sets it on the plate to weight the sauerkraut down.

Nana wipes her hands on her apron and gives the crock a hard look. She wrinkles her brow, purses her lips, and counts on her fingers. "Ten, eleven, twelve. A dozen batches on the scale. Five pounds to a batch. That's sixty pounds. A pint's a pound the world around." She pauses and lifts her eyebrows, glancing toward my mother, with whom she has a long-standing argument on this particular axiom. She is waiting for my mother to point out that a pint of lead does not equal a pint of feathers in pounds. But my mother does not take the bait. She knows the point is moot; the formula works for sauerkraut. So Nana continues her calculations. "Two pints to a quart. Thirty quarts of 'kraut we've got here." And they leave their good day's work to bubble away quietly in the cellar.

꧁꧂

I GREW UP eating sauerkraut throughout the year, cooked with roast pork, heaped on Reuben sandwiches, stirred into baked beans. But if you ask me, the best way to fix it is to start by rendering a few slabs of thick, sliced bacon in a Dutch oven. Pour off the drippings, add a couple of diced onions, a few smashed cloves of garlic, and cook over a low flame until the onions are translucent and the aroma of garlic wafts into the air. Add a quart of sauerkraut—

if it's not homemade, rinse it in water to wash away the extra salt—and break up the strands with the tines of a fork. Should the mood strike you, throw in a grated tart apple, a couple of bay leaves, some cracked black pepper, and a dozen or so juniper berries. A dozen red potatoes, halved or quartered, depending on their size, also make a nice addition. Pour in a healthy dose of white wine and a pint of rich chicken stock. Or not; water will suffice. Put a lid on the pot and simmer the sauerkraut until the potatoes just give way to a knife. Check the pot on occasion, and add more liquid if the sauerkraut seems to be drying out.

Now take some smoked link sausages, something along the lines of bratwurst or knockwurst or Polish sausage, and sear them on all sides in a little oil in a hot skillet—plan on two links per person. Add the links to the sauerkraut and let the kettle simmer for another half-hour. Take the meal to the table and serve it with coarse brown mustard and a heavy round of sourdough rye.

Dish up the sauerkraut and breathe deep the pine scent of juniper, the apple-wood smoke of sausage. Slather mustard on the potatoes and the links, and sop up the juices with hunks torn from the loaf of bread. Wash it down with a glass of dry Reisling or long pulls from a bottle of dark ale. Try to remember as you eat that sauerkraut is not ambrosia of the gods and it is not the latest rage. It is the swill of serfs and farmhands, who sure knew how to dine.

dave's italian kitchen

{ A Y U N H A L L I D A Y }

WHEN I LANDED a job at Dave's Italian Kitchen two
years after graduating from the most expensive university in the
Big Ten, I felt like I'd hit the big time. I'd been running through
restaurants at an alarming rate. I wasn't a very good waitress. I was
slow, I couldn't carry more than three plates at a time, and when
one of my orders got fucked up, I tended to hide in the bathroom
even if the fault lay with the cooks, which it rarely did. A theater
major who gravitated toward anything gauzy and pink, I was miserable in every waitressing uniform I'd heretofore encountered. I
retaliated by rarely washing my apron or the dumpy black pants
I was expected to wear with a white shirt and a tie. I smelled like
salad dressing. My entire life, I have hated salad dressing, even on
salad. Although I made an attempt to pull my long hair back in a
hygienic ponytail, several lank strands always managed to escape,
dangling into my eyes and, occasionally, my mouth. This had been

regarded as a charming character detail when I was making twenty-five dollars an hour posing nude for a figure drawing class, but it infuriated restaurant honchos. This one pompous prick rode me mercilessly about my inability to control my "slovenly" hair. It's a miracle he didn't try to give me bangs with a pair of kitchen shears.

His place was a real nightmare, an overpriced Italian bistro that sold gelato and cappuccino up front during the day. His wife and several of her cronies appeared every lunchtime, laden with shopping bags from upscale boutiques, to hog the window table for hours. They ordered cappuccino and looked at me like there were turds floating in their cups if I failed to froth the milk to their specifications. Under the imperious gaze of Kitty Palucci and her well-heeled pals, I could never get that damn cappuccino machine to work properly. There was no incentive. They never tipped and although they saw me five afternoons a week, they never learned my name, preferring to refer to me as "that girl."

The day shift at Palucci's was pretty slow. Often my only other customer was Palucci's best friend, a commercial theater producer who availed himself of complimentary sundaes and my sub-par cappuccino. He knew I had majored in acting. I always suspected that he was waiting for me to fall to my knees and genuflect before him. In hindsight, this was pure emotional self-defense. He was, after all, a successful theatrical producer and I was a sloppy looking, under-ambitious twenty-three-year-old actress, unwilling to wear makeup or drop the fifteen pounds I couldn't believe I needed to lose before anyone would be willing to send me out on commercial auditions. I consoled myself that this fat cat, who observed Kitty's rule of thumb that a 15 percent gratuity of zero is zero, produced crowd-pleasing schlock like *Steel Magnolias*. In the richly appointed theater of my mind, I starred in the complete works of Shakespeare and Chekhov. In reality, I lurked near the cappuccino machine, glowering behind my unruly strands of hair at those I was fated to serve. Every so often, I ducked below the counter to sneak spoonfuls of gelato, egged on by my fellow café waitress and aspiring actress, Shawna.

Shawna was a diabetic and I indulged her much as Laura Ingalls Wilder helped her blind sister Mary by describing the sights she took in with her own healthy eyes. When it came to gelato, I was Shawna's mouth.

"Hmm, pistachio. I wonder what that would taste like," Shawna would muse, handing me a tasting spoon loaded with three times the amount we were supposed to offer customers.

"Don't you want me to try some of the crème brûlée?" I'd ask, greedily helping myself to another bite.

"*Ooh*, no! It looks like phlegm!" Shawna would reply, loud enough for the customers to hear.

※

DAVE'S ITALIAN KITCHEN didn't have gelato, but that was its only drawback when compared to Palucci's or any of the other twenty-plus restaurants where I had worked, sometimes for no more than a day. For starters, there was the extremely flexible dress code, which Dave had only implemented after repeated customer complaints. The dress code was this: No cutoffs and no bikini tops worn in lieu of shirts. That was it. Once, a new acquaintance was trying to figure out why I looked so familiar. When it came out that she lived in the vicinity of Dave's, I told her that I had worked there for a couple of years. "Oh, Dave's Italian Kitchen!" she laughed. "My husband won't go there. He calls it the place with all the braless waitresses."

You'd think most straight men would enjoy their proximity to a neighborhood institution with legendary spaghetti Carbonara and waitresses who eschew bras, but Dave's was no Hooters. I, for one, always wore a bra, a loose ineffectual one under my sleeveless thrift-store frocks. What I didn't do was shave my armpits and Dave never said a word against it. To this day, he was the best boss I ever had.

⋰⋱

UNLIKE OTHER RESTAURANT managers Dave never seized the opportunity to pump himself up by screaming at an employee who'd undercharged a party of ten or pissed off a table by dropping the entrées they'd been waiting for ever since a certain somebody forgot to turn their ticket in to the cooks an hour ago. Dave never made a big stink. He believed in learning from mistakes, although more than once he inadvertently set me up to make more of them by disrupting my rhythm, which was already syncopated at best. With every table in my section filled, I'd pinwheel around the kitchen, bumping into the more capable waitpersons who appeared like magic to retrieve their orders the second the cooks summoned them. If someone had spilled a puddle of creamy garlic dressing on the tile floor and neglected to mop it up, I could be counted on to slip in it, jettisoning every plate I'd been carrying. Waiters refer to this state as being "in the weeds." Just when I was deepest in the weeds, Dave would summon me over to the pizza ovens, which he manned in a T-shirt, shoveling pies in and out with a long handled wooden paddle.

"Yeah, Dave, what is it?" I gabbled, rifling through my green guest checks in frenzy. I'd be practically panting. "My extra-large half-sausage half-mushroom can't be up yet, can it? I haven't even turned in the ticket. Shit. Sorry. I'm sort of losing it. Whoops, I just heard Jim ringing my bell! Four, that's me, right? I'm coming!"

Dave leaned his forearms on the counter, peeking at me from between stainless-steel shelves filled with cooking utensils and industrial-sized shakers of oregano. "Hey, buddy," he drawled in a resonant baritone, "I was just wondering . . . have you ever read any Evelyn Waugh?"

⁘

DAVE WAS A good man. He was Jewish, not Italian—he had started the business twenty years earlier after a brief stint working for a restaurant supplier. He claimed he'd been appalled at the lengths to which most of the restaurant managers he supplied would go, using only the cheapest, nastiest ingredients to drive their profits up, or, probably more accurately, stand a chance of breaking even. His experience supported what I had seen firsthand in my previous jobs. (One bit of wisdom I like to pass along to people who've never been backstage in a restaurant is never order anything that comes with glazed strawberries. Really. You don't want to know.) Dave harnessed his moral outrage and used it to open his own restaurant, which turned out to be a goldmine. In college, I had steered clear of economics, preferring such useful courses of study as Greek Theatre and Presentational Aesthetics. Dave's Italian Kitchen provided me with the basic education I had eluded for so long, not that I have ever managed to apply the sound business practices that I learned to my own life.

At the outset, Dave had shelled out for an industrial mixer and a pasta cutter, hulking metal contraptions that I feared the way I feared my grandmother's old-fashioned mangle, the one she said would take my arm off if I ventured too close. I was terrified that, skidding on a pat of butter that had tumbled unnoticed from a bread basket, I might pitch head first into the pasta cutter midway through a batch of spinach rotini, or "green noodles" as we called them. "GN" for short. Dave sold these GN and three other proletariat shapes of pasta with several choices of high-cholesterol sauce for unbelievably modest prices. An enormous plate of spaghetti marinara was only $2.95. I rejoiced when every single person at a four-top ordered lasagna because I'd be looking at a minimum tip of three dollars, assuming someone at the table knew how to calculate percentages.

Despite his rock-bottom prices, I always made a lot of moolah at Dave's. On a Saturday night in Section One or Two, a hoary old vet like Gert or Judy could walk out with two hundred fifty bucks easy. As the shift wore on, we stuffed our tips in ricotta buckets with our names scrawled across the side in Magic Marker. At the end of the night, we'd retire to the smoking section one by one to shake our ricotta buckets out over the red-and-white-checked oilcloths, eager to see how our tips measured up against our grand totals. We were honor-bound to tip out 1 percent of our total food sales to the busboys, a much lower amount than is standard restaurant practice. Dave paid them far higher wages than they could have earned bussing anywhere else. At the Kitchen, tipping out was a symbolic act, a show of respect to the guys who had busted their butts alongside us, hauling unappetizing dishpans and resetting the tables while people who'd been waiting in the lobby for twice the host's estimate breathed down their necks. At other places I'd worked, if you had a lousy night, your busboy did too, as his cut was 15 percent of your tips, not 1 percent of however much cheapy-cheap rotini with butter and garlic you'd moved that night. Try handing a busboy seven dollars at the end of a long shift and see how much he loves you.

The busboys at Dave's were all Vietnamese. Many of them were ambitious high-school boys who attended class all day and then worked until almost midnight. They all aspired to emulate Ho, a star waiter who had started out as a busboy. Ho was amazing. He never broke a sweat no matter how many tables the host seated him with simultaneously. I never once saw him in the weeds. He was soft-spoken and neat. Compared to the braless partying waitresses, he was a miracle of discretion.

Besides Ho, who was in a category by himself, there were essentially two tiers to the wait staff. There were the recent college grads like me, people in their early twenties with foolish, romantic degrees and a reasonable chance of knowing who Evelyn Waugh was or, if male, playing in a not-so-good rock band with Dave. We were seen as second-class citizens by the queen bees, Gert and Judy and the rest of their crew who, like the cooks, had started working as teenagers right when the Kitchen first opened. They made the schedules and reported to Dave if someone needed to be fired. The no-bikini-top policy had been put in place in an effort to keep them within the bounds of decency. They ruled the roost, not always with Dave's grace or compassion. In all probability, his magnanimity was only possible because he ceded control of the more pugnacious tasks to these women, tough and loyal townies who weren't afraid to be bitchy. They were excellent waitresses. Manners-wise they could never have cut it in fine dining, but for sheer ability to turn tables, keep their orders straight, and run plates right up their arms from wrist to armpit, they couldn't be beat. They made money hand over fist and ran through it fast. A couple of them were rumored to have impressive drug habits. One time when I asked a cook to help me unclog a drain in the bathroom, he told me to get Gert. "She'll take care of it for you. That nose of hers sucks better than a fucking vacuum cleaner."

Besides the wait staff, the busboys, and the cooks, there was an odd assortment working their way down the ladder in other positions. There were hosts and bartenders, aspiring waiters whose job it was to sell seventy-five cent glasses of wine-in-a-box to the testy crowd in the small holding pen that passed for a lobby. Dave never advertised, but from the time the doors opened at 4:30 in the afternoon, the place was packed. The people waiting to be seated had a clear view past the host and bartender into the kitchen, where we non-veteran waiters sneaked bites of our customers' leftover chicken Marsala before wrapping the remaining portion to go. This gross violation of health codes made little sense, since Dave let us order practically anything we wanted from the menu for free, four dollars for chicken or veal. The only thing he asked us not to eat was the chocolate mousse, which was stored in a non-industrial refrigerator at the back of the dining room, where the soda and coffee dispensers were. It was not uncommon for a customer searching for the john to stumble across a waitress crouched behind the refrigerator's open door, pile-driving chocolate mousse. We also piped cannoli filling straight from the bag into our gaping maws, again in full view of the throng wedged into the tiny lobby.

⁘

I BECAME VERY proud of my identity as a waitress, now that I no longer had to wear a sexless black-and-white uniform and get stiffed making cappuccinos for the boss's wife. Dave's didn't even have a cappuccino machine, though we did have our share of troublemaking customers. There was a repellent couple named, I swear to god, the Piggies. The Piggies had been eating at Dave's once a week since it opened and of course they thought they owned the joint. Gert or Judy would greet them like royalty at the door only to pawn them off immediately on me or Issac, a great disappointment to the Piggies. They knew about the hierarchy of the waiters. Issac and I were artsy college kids. We wouldn't last more than a couple of years. Gert and Judy were there for the duration. The Piggies could only be seated at Booth Six, a prime bit of real estate that could easily accommodate a large party of prime tippers who would eat and get out. The Piggies liked their food prepared in certain ways depending on who was cooking that night. They'd detain me forever, forcing me to recite their order back to them, suspicious that a rookie would never be able to remember all their little nuances and pet peeves. I tried to smile reassuringly, which only seemed to aggravate them further. Meanwhile, I could hear the cooks pounding on the bell and roaring my name as orders I'd placed backed up on the counter.

Once, Mrs. Piggie tasted her manicotti and puckered her already tight mouth. "I can't eat this. There's no way Jim cooked this. Take it back and tell them I want Jim to cook it."

I carried the plate into the kitchen and told Jim, who had cooked it, what Mrs. Piggie had said. Jim, a taciturn long-suffering man who was engaged to marry the perkiest of the veteran waitresses, rolled his eyes and shoved it back in the oven.

"She says she likes it brown on—"

"I know. I know. Brown on the edges, but not too brown, with just enough sauce, whatever that means. Fucking Piggies." Jim rolled the manicotti onto a fresh plate and sent me back to Booth Six.

Without so much as a grunt of appreciation, Mrs. Piggie forked up a small bite and yipped like a Yorkshire terrier who's just realized he's been poisoned. "No! This is all wrong! Did you tell Jim it's for me? Honestly!"

She flung herself back against the tall wooden booth, glaring at her husband with hostility, as if to say, "Well, what can you expect from these new people?" Issac, uncorking a bottle of wine at a table across the way, shot me a sympathetic look.

Back in the kitchen, Jim stonewalled, refusing to tinker any further with the manicotti or prepare anything else for Mrs. Piggie to eat that evening. I pleaded to no avail. Finally, one of the other cooks, a loose cannon named Tommy, reached across to snatch the plate out of my hands. "Gimme that!" he shouted, throwing the manicotti into a hot pan with an entire stick of butter. He knocked them around with a wooden spoon for a couple of seconds, spit in the pan and re-plated the offending dish yet again with a fresh ladle's worth of meat sauce. "There! Give that to the old bitch and make sure she eats every bite! Tell her that Jim cooked it!"

I did as instructed and anyone who has ever worked in a restaurant will be glad if hardly surprised to learn that Mrs. Piggie cleaned her plate on this third attempt, cooing contentedly over the special treatment "Jim" had lavished on her.

·❖·

THE WALLS OF Dave's Italian Kitchen were lined with testaments to the abiding power of love. Parties who finished a bottle of wine could autograph the dead soldier's label and give it to their waiter to stick on the ledge that ran around the dining room just above eye level. There it would remain for eternity—or at least until another starry-eyed drunken couple sent their bottle up to replace it. Besides the fresh daisies on the red-and-white tablecloths and some terrifying abstract acrylics by one of the delivery guys, the bottles were the only attempt at decoration. It was another genius move on Dave's part, a way to ensure that he'd move some higher-ticket vino along with the stuff that flew out of the box for cheap.

Once, when the Bulls were in the playoffs or the Bears were winning the Superbowl or something of that magnitude was keeping the customers away, a waitress named Drake-Ann and I amused ourselves by reading the dusty bottles, looking for the names of people we knew. I recognized lots of friends from college, sometimes wondering why I hadn't been invited to join the boisterous parties of six who'd signed their Chianti bottles in such Falstaffian merriment. While I was thus ruminating, Drake-Ann fished her pen out of her apron and scrawled something on a bottle.

"Drake-Ann, what are you doing?" I hissed, scandalized.

Flashing her engaging, irresponsible smile, she passed the bottle over for my inspection. I squinted at the label:

Michael and Debbie got engaged at Dave's Italian Kitchen on April 14, 1982. Love you forever.

P.S.—Drake-Ann was here too.

I couldn't believe she had breached the sanctity of the bottles.

"Oh, come on! Who do you think ever looks at those old things?" she taunted, holding her pen up for me to take. Shaking my head, I glanced around to make sure we were unobserved. I wondered what Gert would say to Dave if she caught us at this asinine prank, horning in on other people's long-gone good times. I wanted to bond with her, so I shrugged and wrote:

I was also here. Congratulations Mike + Debbie! Love 4ever, Ayun Halliday

---

WE SKIPPED AROUND the dining room, embellishing bottles at random until the game grew weary.

Several weeks later, I saw a couple in my section take a bottle off the ledge and hold it up to the light. Uh-oh. I wished I'd never let Drake-Ann pressure me into that stupid trick. What if I'd signed their special bottle, thinking I was so funny? What if they complained to the manager? Worried, I dove into the kitchen to collect an order that was up for another of my tables. When I returned, they both had bottles in each hand, shaking them like maracas. I hurried over.

"Can I, uh, get you anything else?" I asked.

"Take a look," the man said, offering one of his bottles. His girl-friend made small fascinated grunts as she continued to rattle hers. Were they stoned? What they were, it turns out, was revolted. I could see why. At the bottom of the bottle, six legs pointing stiffly toward the ceiling, was a dead cockroach. People at the surrounding tables, their curiosity piqued by this couple's antics, were reaching for the bottles nearest them. A quick visual check revealed that every bottle on the ledge boasted at least one cancelled *cucaracha*.

I darted into the kitchen to alert the boss. "Dave! Dave! We've got a problem! Everybody in my section is shaking the bottles! They're all full of roaches, dead roaches!"

"Oh gnarly!" Tommy the cook cried happily. "It must've been the exterminator! The exterminator was here yesterday fogging for bugs. That's so fucking gross!"

Dave sighed and wiped his hands on his T-shirt before stretching another lump of pizza dough to fit the pan. "Well, buddy, what do you suggest I do about it?"

"I don't know! Can I offer them a free chocolate mousse or something?"

"Sure, buddy, if that's what you want," Dave mumbled, no doubt realizing that for every mousse I comped a customer, I'd help myself to two.

❖

I MISS DAVE'S. I miss the money, finding crumpled twenties in my pockets every time I did the laundry. I miss the checkered tablecloths and the bottles, which were recycled the morning after we discovered the roaches. I miss the phone numbers scrawled on the kitchen walls and waiting on other waiters. I don't miss the Piggies, nor do I miss the sauce-cheeked toddlers who threw grubby handfuls of cut-up spaghetti onto the brown industrial carpeting beneath Booth Eleven. Now I take my own young children to restaurants, hoping my broad smile telegraphs the juicy tip with which I plan to counteract the annoyance I've visited on the establishment. Often since becoming a mother, I've revisited that sensation of being in the weeds, as well as the never-ending side work. I can still carry three plates on my arm, but in the domestic setting, this number seems impressive. More than anything else, I miss the sense of absolute freedom that came when I boarded the El at one in the morning, reeking of sweat and creamy garlic dressing, a wad of cash in my bra and a large free-of-charge pizza in the box on my lap. One night, a drunk homeless guy teasingly asked me for a slice. To his surprise, I lifted the lid and invited all our fellow

passengers to help themselves. I have never felt more professionally powerful than I did in that moment, even though the homeless guy wrinkled his nose when he saw the anchovies.

Note from the Editor

WHEN I WAS compiling essays for *Women Who Eat,* Kate Sekules, one of the contributors, suggested I contact her friend, writer Amanda Davis, to see whether she'd like to write something for the book. I knew that Amanda, author of *Wonder When You'll Miss Me* and *Circling the Drain: Stories,* was a wonderful writer, and I jumped at the chance.

We played email and phone tag for a few weeks and finally I reached Amanda at home. She was enthusiastic about the project and said yes, she definitely wanted to write a piece. She'd been mulling over an idea for her essay, she said, about leaving vegetarianism after seventeen years of not eating meat. I was intrigued—I was a vegetarian for twelve years myself, and started eating just sausage first, then everything. I still feel the guilt, I told her. "Can I ask," I said hesitantly, "why? How?"

"I was in a yoga class," she said, "and suddenly, I just needed meat. I still don't know why. But I got up from the floor, grabbed my things and walked out. I kept walking, straight to Balducci's and said to the woman behind the counter, 'Can you help me? I've never done this before.' I had no idea how much I should order. I bought bloody, rare roast beef and ate it right then. After that all I wanted was the rarest meat. The funniest thing is since I hadn't eaten meat in so long, the texture of it was so apparent to me. It was so clear I was eating *flesh*. I still think eating chicken feels like chewing someone's arm."

⸪

TWO DAYS BEFORE Amanda's essay was due, she was killed in a plane crash while on book tour. I'm sorry not to be able to publish her essay here, and I'm sorry a fine writer and a really lovely woman are lost to us now. But I'll never forget the story Amanda told me that day. Now maybe you won't either.

Contributor Biographies

Josie Aaronson-Gelb is pursuing an MFA in writing at the University of Montana. She is the author of "Gastronomically Correct," a food column that ran for a year in the *Oakland Tribune* and for two years at Cornell University. Her other work has appeared in *Nation's Restaurant News*, *San Francisco Magazine* and *Pegasus* Magazine. She was a finalist in the televised cooking competition Master Chef USA and has cooked professionally in several Northern California restaurants. She spent four years at Cornell University attending the School of Hotel Management but her true love is cooking large-scale dinner parties for her friends—as long as they do the dishes.

Faith Adiele was raised in the Pacific Northwest on trout she caught with her Swedish-American grandfather and limpa bread she baked with her Finnish-American grandmother. When she was fifteen, she began traveling to countries with spices—Mexico, Thailand—to satisfy her other half, and at age twenty-six, she went to Nigeria to find her father and siblings. These cultural journeys have been chronicled in such publications as *Essence, Ms., A Woman Alone* (Seal Press), and *Her Fork in the Road* (Travelers' Tales), and are the subject of a PBS documentary, "The Journey Home." Her memoir, "Meeting Faith: The Forest Journals of a Black Buddhist Nun," is due from Norton in 2004. She is Assistant Professor of Creative Writing at the University of Pittsburgh.

Marianne Apostolides is the author of *Inner Hunger: A Young Woman's Struggle Through Anorexia and Bulimia,* published by W.W. Norton. She is currently writing her second book of literary nonfiction, as well as mothering her two children, Athanasia and Romeo. Peanut butter on toast, after her children are asleep, has become an important part of her daily diet. She lives in Toronto.

Christine Basham is a mother of four and former missionary to Thailand. Now a heathen freelance writer, an older and wiser Ms. Basham writes from her home in Maryland. Her foodie ramblings appear in *A Cup of Comfort Cookbook,* and the soon-to-be-published "A Royal Fork Up: 101 of the Worst Recipe Blunders Ever."

Seattle-based freelance writer **Kate Chynoweth** covers good parties, bad dresses, and etiquette in her book *The Bridesmaid Guide* (Chronicle Books) and food history, lore, and cooking in her book *Lemons* (Chronicle Books). She is also the editor of the forthcoming Northern California and Pacific Northwest volumes of the *Best Places to Kiss* guidebook series (Sasquatch

Books). Her writing on food, travel, and lifestyle appears in *Sunset, Seattle* magazine, and other magazines.

Camille Cusumano is the author of several cookbooks, including *Rodale's Basic Natural Foods Cookbook* (co-writer), *The New Foods* (Henry Holt), and *America Loves Salads* (Doubleday), and has written articles on food, fitness, and travel for many publications, including the *New York Times, San Francisco Chronicle, Los Angeles Times, Islands Magazine*, and *Country Living*. She published her first novel, *The Last Cannoli*, a runner-up for the James Jones First Novel Fellowship, in 2000 (Legas). She is a senior editor at *VIA* magazine in San Francisco.

Karen Eng edits and publishes *PekoPeko: a zine about food* (www.pekopekozine.com). A freelance writer and editor, she has worked in both independent and mainstream national magazines since 1991. In 2002 she received a George Washington Williams journalism fellowship sponsored by the Independent Press Association. Current projects include editing a book about friendships between women, forthcoming by Seal Press, as well as a *PekoPeko* omnibus. She lives in England.

Rachel Fudge has her fingers in many pies, none of which is actually edible. A grammarian by trade and by nature, she is also an editor at *Bitch* magazine and a freelance writer for such fine independent publications as *PekoPeko, Arcane,* and *Nebulosi*. She lives and drinks in San Francisco with her special peer, Hugh, who mixes a very fine martini.

Kara Gall, a.k.a. Loam Akasha-Bast, is a recovering sausage-tarian. Although she is heiress to over 1,400 acres of land in Nebraska, she currently lives with her daughter in a small, overpriced apartment in the San Francisco Bay Area. The editor of *inFlame Magazine,* her writing has appeared in San Francisco's *Reclaiming Quarterly* and the anthologies *Breeder* and *ReGeneration.* Visit her online at www.kybela.com

Alisa Gordaneer lives and writes in Victoria, B.C., Canada, where she's the editor of *Monday Magazine,* Victoria's alternative newsweekly, and the mother of two small kids. Her work has appeared in *Threshold* (Sono Nis), *Love and Pomegranates* (Sono Nis), *Breeder* (Seal Press, 2001), and a variety of periodicals.

Ayun Halliday is the sole staff member of the quarterly zine *The East Village Inky,* the 2002 Firecracker Alternative Book Award winner for best zine. Her first book, *The Big Rumpus: A Mother's Tale from the Trenches* was published by Seal Press in 2002, and her second, *No Touch Monkey! And Other Travel Lessons Learned Too Late* (Seal Press) is on shelves now. She is a frequent contributor to *BUST* and *Hip Mama* and her essays have appeared in the anthologies *Breeder, A Woman Alone,* and *The Unsavvy Traveler.* As a member of the Neo-Futurists, she wrote and performed in several full-length solo works as well as hundreds of short plays for *Too Much Light Makes the Baby Go Blind (30 Plays in 60 Minutes).* She lives in Brooklyn with her children and husband, the man responsible for *Urinetown (The Musical).* More at www.ayunhalliday.com.

Suzanne Hamlin coedited *The Best American Recipes 1999* and *2000,* and is a writer for the *New York Times.* She founded the *New York Daily News* Food Section and writes for national magazines. Hamlin also coordinates the annual workshop for food writers and editors at the Culinary Institute of America at Greystone in St. Helena, California.

contributor biographies

Christina Henry de Tessan is an editor in San Francisco. She is the editor of *Expat: Women's True Tales of Life Abroad* and coeditor of *A Woman Alone: Travel Tales from around the Globe*, both published by Seal Press, and author of the "Paris City Walks" Deck (forthcoming from Chronicle Books).

Amanda Hesser is a food reporter at the *New York Times*, and wrote the "Food Diary" column for the *New York Times Magazine*. She is the author of *The Cook and the Gardener* and *Cooking for Mr. Latte*, both published by W. W. Norton & Company. Recipient of the Literary Food Writing Award, she lives with her husband in Brooklyn Heights, New York.

Lisa Jervis is the editor and publisher of *Bitch: Feminist Response to Pop Culture*. A transplanted New Yorker, she lives in Oakland, California, with two cats, a six-quart KitchenAid mixer, and a strong desire for two ovens that can only be satisfied by knocking out the only closet in her house. She is seriously considering it.

Theresa Lust has worked in restaurants from the Pacific Northwest to New England, and is the author of *Pass the Polenta*. She lives in New Hampshire with her husband.

Pooja Makhijani is a graduate of Johns Hopkins University where she received her degree in Biomedical Engineering. As a freelance journalist, her bylines have appeared in the *New York Times,* the *Village Voice,* the *Newark Star-Ledger,* the *Indian Express, Time Out New York, NY ARTS Magazine,* and *India Today* among others and her essays have appeared in *Bibi* and *Cicada*. In addition, she has taught classes in writing and publishing at Middlesex County College in Edison, New Jersey. Makhijani is now a student in the MFA (Writing) Program at Sarah Lawrence College in Bronxville, New York.

Debra Meadow is a freelance journalist and visual artist from Portland, Oregon. She writes for local Portland papers such as the *Tribune* and the *Southwest Community Connection,* where she does a monthly feature on art and artists as well as other feature articles. Her artwork encompasses varied media, including oil and acrylic paints and collage, pieced fabric, and photography. She is currently working on a novel.

Lela Nargi is a writer and freelance reporter who lives in Brooklyn, New York. Her essays appear in *Natural Bridge, Gastronomica, Descant, Hotel Amerika,* and *The Raven Chronicles.* Her essay "Into the Thar" was listed in the Notables section of *Best American Travel Writing 2002.* She is the author of *All U Can Eat,* a cookbook for beginners, *Knitting Lessons: Tales from the Knitting Path,* and is working on an untitled book about women and food. She has worked for such publications as *People, Life, Entertainment Weekly,* and *House & Garden,* and she currently contributes articles on art, photography, and culture to a variety of national and international magazines.

Elizabeth Nunez is a CUNY Distinguished Professor at Medgar Evers College, New York. The author of five novels— *Grace, Discretion, Bruised Hibiscus, Beyond the Limbo Silence,* and *When Rocks Dance*—she lives in Amityville, New York. Visit www.elizabethnunez.com for more information.

Terez Rose has lived in London as well as Africa, and has really good recipes for sticky toffee pudding and spicy peanut soup. Her work has appeared in the *San Jose Mercury News,* the

Milwaukee Journal-Sentinel, the Spokane *Spokesman-Review, Peace Corps Online,* and *Big World* travel magazine. She makes her home with husband and son in California's Santa Cruz Mountains, where mother and son fight regularly over frozen versus organic. She is currently seeking representation for her novel, "Black Ivory Soul," and would love to hear from you at terez.rose@ sbcglobal.net.

Kate Sekules is the travel editor of *Food & Wine* magazine, and the author of *The Boxer's Heart: Lessons from the Ring.* She lives with her family in Brooklyn.

Christine Sienkiewicz is a writer and book designer and a contributor to *Kitchen Sink* magazine. She has also written for *Fabula* magazine and Hesperian health publications. She lives in San Francisco with her husband.

Cheryl Strayed is the author of the novel *TORCH,* which is set in rural northern Minnesota, where she grew up. Her fiction and memoir have been published in *DoubleTake, Nerve,* and *The Sun,* among other magazines, and in several anthologies, most notably *The Best New American Voices 2003* and twice in *The Best American Essays.* A graduate of the University of Minnesota and Syracuse University, she currently lives in Portland, Oregon, where she is at work on a book-length memoir.

Amanda Sullivan is a former actress with a master's degree in gender politics from NYU. She currently divides her time between her business—The Perfect Daughter: Chaos Control— and caring for her son, Henry. She is looking forward to Henry's third birthday party, for which she has an excellent menu planned.

contributor biographies

Stephanie Susnjara is a freelance writer whose essays have appeared in *Brain, Child* and *The Yorkville Anthology of New Writers.* She lives in New York City with her husband and their two children.

Michelle Tea is the author of *The Passionate Mistakes and Intricate Corruption of One Girl in America*, the award-winning *Valencia,* and a Lambda-nominated memoir, *The Chelsea Whistle.* She is currently editing a book on working-class women called "Without a Net" that is forthcoming with Seal Press. Tea lives in San Francisco.

Gretchen VanEsselstyn has been eating food since the early seventies. Her work has appeared on various websites and on tables across the tri-state area. Gretchen lives in Brooklyn, New York. She can kill a lobster with her bare hands.

About the Editor

Leslie Miller is the senior editor of Seal Press. Her essays and stories have appeared in numerous anthologies and other publications, including *The Unsavvy Traveler, Young Wives' Tales,* and *Bare Your Soul.* Currently at work on her first novel, she lives and cooks with her family in Seattle.

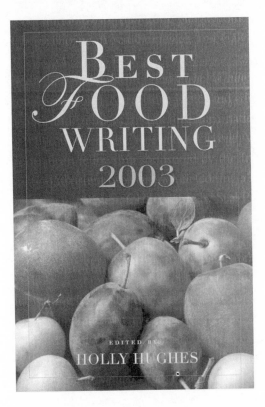

The fourth edition of this annual collection assembles the most exceptional writing from the past year's books, magazines, newspapers, newsletters, and websites. Read our best writers on everything from the intricacies of the restaurant business to re-creating one's favorite childhood treats. Including pieces from such stars of the genre as John Thorne, Amanda Hesser, and Calvin Trillin.

Praise for a past edition of Best Food Writing:

"Hughes serves up this year's offering like a satisfying, well-rounded meal."—*Publishers Weekly*

Published by Marlowe & Co.
ISBN 1-56924-440-5
Available at your local bookstore.